Allied Health Professions—Essential Guides

Key Tools and Techniques in management and leadership of the Allied Health Professions

Robert Jones

and

Fiona Jenkins

Series Foreword by
Penny Humphris

Foreword by
Jim Easton

Radcliffe Publishing Ltd
London • New York

Radcliffe Publishing Ltd
70 Alston Drive
Bradwell Abbey
Milton Keynes
MK13 9HG
United Kingdom

www.radcliffepublishing.com

Electronic catalogue and worldwide online ordering facility.

British Library Cataloguing in Publication Data

A catalogue record for this book is available from the British Library.

ISBN-13: 978 184619 532 7

The paper used for the text pages of this book is FSC certified. FSC (The Forest Stewardship Council) is an international network to promote responsible management of the world's forests.

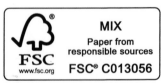

Typeset by KnowledgeWorks Global Ltd, Chennai, India
Cover design by Cox Design Ltd, Witney, Oxon, UK
Printed and bound by TJI Digital, Padstow, Cornwall, UK

Contents

List of figures   ix
List of tables   xi
List of boxes   xii
CD contents   xiv
Series foreword   xv
Foreword   xvii
Preface   xix
About the authors   xxi
List of contributors   xxiii
List of abbreviations   xxv
List of templates   xxix
List of books in this series   xxxi

1 Allied Health Professions' Management Quality Matrix   **1**
Fiona Jenkins and Robert Jones
Introduction   1
Metrics   2
Key performance indicators (KPIs)   3
Business performance management (BPM)   3
Lean thinking   3
Six Sigma   4
Total quality management   5
Benefits realisation   6
Clinical dashboard   7
Balanced scorecard   7
AHP management quality matrix   8
Strategy   10
Patient and service user experience   11
Clinical excellence   13

Finance   14
Information and metrics   16
Activity   17
Staff resource effectiveness   19
Staff management and development   20
Service improvement and redesign   21
Leadership and management development   23
Risk management   24
Corporate governance   25
Communications and marketing   26
Key performance indicators   28
References   29

2 **Assessment tool for evaluating AHP management structures** **31**
   Fiona Jenkins and Robert Jones
   Introduction   31
   Application of the *Tool*   32
   Scoring system: assessment Tool for AHP management models 33
   Conclusion   33
   Strategic management   34
   Clinical governance   37
   Human resource management   38
   Clinical/professional requirements   39
   Operational/service management   41
   Resource management   42
   Information management   43
   Education   44
   Commissioning   45
   Service improvement/modernisation   46

3 **Benchmarking AHP services**   **49**
   Fiona Jenkins and Robert Jones
   Benchmarking your service   49
   Introducing our AHP benchmarking tool   49
   How to use the tool   50
   The benchmarking 'toolkit'   50
   Briefing notes   50
   Section 1 your organisation—general information   52
   Section 2 your professional group and staffing   52
   Section 3 inpatient services   55
   Section 4 outpatient services   55
   Section 5 community services   57
   Reference   59

4 **Time is money—how do we spend it? Analysing staff activity**   **61**
Robert Jones and Fiona Jenkins
Introduction   61
Tips for implementation   62
Therapy services activity sample *pro forma*   64
Example of reports from activity sample   65

5 **Principles for computerised information systems for**
   AHP services   **69**
Robert Jones and Fiona Jenkins
Introduction   69
Principles for computerised information systems for AHP services   70

6 **Functions for Allied Health Professions' record systems**   **73**
Margaret Hastings
Information management   73

7 **Using the Myers-Briggs Type Indicator within the allied**
   health professions   **77**
Simon and Sheena Loveday
Introduction   77
Five scenarios   78
Background to the indicator   78
Type and preference   79
The four dimensions of type   80
How do you take it forward?   87
References   88
Further reading   88

8 **Appraisal: 360° feedback**   **89**
Simon and Sheena Loveday
Introduction: what is 360° feedback? And what is the point of
gathering it?   89
So why use this process?   90
Putting it into practice: choosing the right method   91
How to gather the feedback   92
What questions to ask   93
Who (and how many) to ask   95
Briefing your respondents   95
Using other instruments   96
Receiving the feedback   97
Receiving feedback—or checking it out—face-to-face   98
So what next—how do you follow up?   99
References   99

9 Four basic behavioural styles   **101**
Anne Mandy and Gail Louw
Introduction   101
Strengths and weaknesses of each style   103
Styles within teams and organisations   103
Communication styles of each category   104
References   106

10 Adult learning and self-directed learners   **107**
Kay Mohanna, Elizabeth Cottrell, David Wall, and Ruth Chambers
Introduction   107
T1/S4 mismatch   109
T1/S3–S4 mismatch   109
T4/S1 mismatch   110
The false Stage 4 learner   111
Dependent, resistant learners as a product of the educational
system   111
Using the SSDL model in practice   111
Brookfield's principles of adult learning   112
How to put the principles of adult learning into practice   112
Work-based learning   113
References   118

11 Developing your teaching style and techniques   **119**
Kay Mohanna, Elizabeth Cottrell, David Wall, and Ruth Chambers
Introduction   119
Be aware of your own teaching style(s)   119
Investigate your teaching style   120
Step 1: work out your preferred teaching style(s) by answering the
following questions   121
Step 2: complete your scoring grid   122
Step 3: rate each teaching style   123
Step 4: plot your preferred teaching style(s) on the sets hexagon   123
Tailoring your teaching style(s) to students' learning style(s)   124
Matching your teaching style to learners' needs and preferences   125
Mismatch between teaching style and stage of learning   126
References   128
Further reading   128

12 Models, techniques, and approaches for change management 129
Robert Jones and Fiona Jenkins
Introduction   129
Change   130
Key concepts   131
Culture   133
Leadership   134
Teams   136
Models, techniques, and approaches for
change management   136
Communicating change   143
Change leadership   144
How to overcome 'change fatigue'   144
Critical mistakes and errors   146
Key factors in effective change management   146
Key behaviours and success factors   147
Framework for the management of change   148
Case study 'choice appointments'   150
Moving from the current to the desired situation   150
Essential actions   151
Skills for success   153
Evaluation   154
Learning points   157
Conclusions   158
Conclusion–change management   158
References   160

13 Outcome measurement Matrix for AHP services   163
Robert Jones and Fiona Jenkins
Introduction   163
Outcome Measures for Outpatient Services   164
Effectiveness score   165
Efficiency score   165
Outcome measurement Matrix   165
Outcome measures: inpatient services   167
Outcome measures: community domiciliary   168
Using the Matrix flexibly   169
Recording outcome measures   169
References   169

14 Care pathways and the Allied Health Professional   **171**
Fiona Jenkins and Robert Jones
The link between AHPs and care pathways   171
What is a care pathway   172
The history and spread of care pathways   174
Why develop care pathways?   174
What care pathways contain   175
Care pathways and clinical governance   175
The aim of care pathways   176
Ten phases to developing care pathways   178
Evaluation of care pathways   192
The purpose of analysis and review   193
How to use care pathways   194
Benefits and barriers   194
Conclusion   195
References   196
Further reading   197

15 Top tips for report writing   **199**
Fiona Jenkins and Robert Jones
Checklist for report writing   199

16 Top tips for report presentation   **201**
Robert Jones and Fiona Jenkins
Checklist for report presentation   201

17 Templates   **205**
Robert Jones and Fiona Jenkins
17.1 AHP Clinical governance reporting   206
17.2 AHP services human resources reports   215
17.3 Example AHP activity report   224

18 Useful guidance   **225**
Robert Jones and Fiona Jenkins
Using time effectively   225
The seven principles of public life   227
'The rules that stifle change that MUST be broken'   228
Is everyone the architect of their own future?   228

List of figures

Figure 4.1: Sub-division of staff time by staff band

Figure 4.2: Sub-division of staff time; all staff

Figure 4.3: Comparison of outpatient staff: patient-related to non-patient-related activity by Band 5 and Band 7, physiotherapy outpatient service

Figure 8.1: Feedback grid

Figure 9.1: The strengths and weaknesses of each behavioural style adapted from Bolton and Bolton

Figure 10.1: Adult learning and self-directed learners

Figure 11.1: Your preferred teaching style(s)

Figure 12.1: Learning dip and sigmoid curve

Figure 12.2: A hierarchy of leadership

Figure 12.3: An overview of change management tools, models, and approaches

Figure 12.4: Reactions to change

Figure 12.5: Iceberg process

Figure 12.6: Force field analysis

Figure 12.7: PDSA cycle

Figure 12.8: SWOT analysis

Figure 12.9: PEST analysis

Figure 12.10: Percentage DNA

Figure 12.11: Routine waiting time

Figure 12.12: Waiting time complaints

Figure 12.13: Was the information provided by the physiotherapy service appointment system clear

Figure 12.14: Would any other information have been useful?

Figure 13.1: Outcome measurement Matrix—example 1

Figure 13.2: Outcome measurement Matrix—example 2

Figure 13.3: Outcome measurement Matrix—inpatients

Figure 13.4: Outcome measurement Matrix—inpatients—example 3

Figure 14.1: Integrated care pathways and clinical governance

Figure 14.2: Plan do study act cycle—adapted from Langley et al

Figure 14.3: An example of an ICP algorithm for Parkinson's disease.

Figure 14.4: An example of an algorithm for back pain.

Figure 14.5: An example of patient produced information.

Figure 14.6: Patient version of care pathway.

Figure 14.7: A care pathway continuous cycle of improvement.

List of tables

Table 2.1:   Completed example template of assessment tool
Table 2.2:   Assessment of management structures: the assessment tool
Table 3.1:   Spreadsheet 1: your organisation
Table 3.2:   Spreadsheet 2: your professional group
Table 3.3:   Spreadsheet 3: inpatient services
Table 3.4:   Spreadsheet 4: outpatient services
Table 3.5:   Spreadsheet 5: community services
Table 6.1:   Functions for record systems to support AHP clinical recording
Table 8.1:   Belbin Shaper role
Table 9.1:   Communication styles, limitations, and most preferred electronic communication style
Table 10.1: Stages of development of learning and teaching, leading to self-directed learning
Table 10.2: Mismatch of levels of self-direction of learning with type of delivery of teaching
Table 11.1: Teaching delivery matched against the six SETS teaching styles
Table 12.1: Seven phases to social change intervention
Table 12.2: Change leadership
Table 12.3: Leading change—why transformation efforts fail
Table 12.4: Change management factors
Table 12.5: Key behaviours and success factors

List of boxes

Box 1.1:   Questions to ask to eliminate waste
Box 1.2:   Six Sigma DMAIC process
Box 1.3:   Key elements of TQM
Box 1.4:   Five major features of clinical dashboards
Box 1.5:   Reasons for implementing the balanced scorecard approach
Box 1.6:   The 14 AHP Management Quality Standards
Box 4.1:   Therapy services activity sample form: briefing notes
Box 8.1:   Preliminary questionnaire
Box 8.2:   Self-dialogue
Box 9.1:   Categories of behavioural style
Box 10.1: Knowles' guidelines on teaching self-directed adults
Box 10.2: How to create an adult learner
Box 10.3: Tips from experienced teachers
Box 11.1: Tips from experienced teachers
Box 12.1: Processes for development
Box 12.2: Eight-stage process of change
Box 12.3: Communication strategy
Box 12.4: Framework for the management of change
Box 12.5: Reactions to change
Box 13.1: Effectiveness scoring
Box 14.1: NPA definition of a care pathway
Box 14.2: The aims of care pathways
Box 14.3: Ten phases to developing care pathways
Box 14.4: Project team members and skills
Box 14.5: Types of key indicators
Box 14.6: Items for consideration when developing ICP documentation
Box 14.7: Checklist for pathway maintenance
Box 14.8: Benefits and barriers to care pathway implementation
Box 15.1: Checklist for report writing
Box 16.1: Checklist for report presentation

Box 18.1: Some tips for managing your time effectively
Box 18.2: The seven principles of public life
Box 18.3: Key aspirations

CD contents

AHP management quality matrix (*pp.* 10–29)
Assessment tool for evaluating AHP management structures (*pp.* 34–47)
The benchmarking 'toolkit' (*pp.* 51, 53, 54, 56, 58)
Therapy services activity sample *pro forma* (*pp.* 64–65)
Outcome measurement Matrix for AHP services (*pp.* 163–169)
Templates (*pp.* 206–224)

Series foreword

The NHS, the biggest organisation in the UK and reputedly the third largest in the world, is undergoing massive transformation. We know that effective leadership is essential if the health service is to achieve continuous improvement in the services it offers. It needs people from all types of backgrounds—clinical and managerial—to step up and take on leadership roles to shape the future of health improvement and healthcare delivery.

Leaders are needed at every level of the health service. The concept of leadership only coming from the top and being defined by position and title is now out of date. It is much more about ways of thinking and behaving and individuals seeing themselves as having the potential to make a real difference for patients. Effective leadership is about working in partnerships and teams to develop a vision for the future, set the direction, influence those whose input is needed and deliver results—a high quality, safe, timely, and accessible health service for all.

Allied health professionals operate in every setting in which healthcare is delivered. You have unparalleled opportunities to help patients to lead their own care and to see how services to patients, clients, and carers can be improved across entire patient pathways, crossing traditional professional and organisational boundaries to improve patients' experiences. You have the potential to make a difference by leading improvement and managing services and resources well.

There are already many outstanding leaders in the NHS in the allied health professions making a real difference to services. Two of them had the vision for this series of books and have worked with formidable energy and commitment to make them a reality. Robert and Fiona have both made a considerable investment in their own professional and personal development and delivered substantial improvements in the services for which they are responsible. They have increased their awareness, skills, and knowledge and taken on leadership roles, putting into practice many of their ideas and learning. They have worked tirelessly to spread their learning and skilfully persuaded a great many academics and practitioners to contribute to these books to provide a rich collection of theories, tools, techniques, and insights to help you.

This series of books has been written to encourage and support many more of you to embark on or to continue your development, to enhance your leadership and management skills, knowledge, and experience, and to give you confidence to take on new roles and responsibilities. I am sure that many of you, who have not previously considered yourselves as leaders will, when you have read these books, reconsider your roles and potential and take the next steps on your journeys.

Penny Humphris, former Director of the NHS Leadership Centre

May 2011

Foreword

The NHS is facing the greatest period of challenge in its history. Firstly, from the need to continue to sustain and improve quality against a period of significant economic stringency. Secondly, in implementing wide-ranging reforms designed to put patients and clinicians at the heart of decision-making. The key to success in both these challenges is, of course, leadership.

Allied Health Professionals will be a central part of this leadership response. Leading the redesign of key patient pathways; supporting the work to keep patients well and out of hospital, and to leave hospital earlier and fitter; and supporting the commissioning process. For Allied Health Professionals, this is both a challenge and an opportunity. In this work, Robert and Fiona continue their series supporting Allied Health Professionals in that leadership journey. It is an important contribution to this critical effort.

Jim Easton
NHS National Director for Improvement and Efficiency
May 2011

Preface

When we first had the idea of writing and editing a series of books specifically for Allied Health Professions' managers, leaders, clinicians, educators, and researchers and a wide range of other disciplines in healthcare, one of our guiding principles was based on the question: What books would have been useful to us when we first 'landed' management and leadership or senior clinical roles? How could we support colleagues in these roles, and what might be useful to them in the AHP services or in other disciplines within the NHS? We also thought about what might be a positive contribution to the wider healthcare management and leadership literature, help others to understand the background and remit of AHP services, wanting to improve awareness of what we do, who we are, where we are 'coming from', and about where we want to be and what our aspirations are for patient care, our staff, the organisations we work in, and the wider community.

We wanted to provide positive, inspirational, and useful material for our colleagues, to incorporate others who have great expertise and experience in their own fields, and to share our own work and experience to help and support AHPs by providing a 'tried and tested' evidence base. Perhaps in a small way we could help set the direction, or at least reflect 'best' practice. In our experience, there was very little in the literature, certainly not much written from and for a specific Allied Health Professions angle.

As we move ever more deeply into the fiscal 'ice age' and the future healthcare agenda encompasses growing scarcity in an era of growth of demand, or to put it another way; infinite demand, finite resources, we must be positive about maximising our managerial and clinical effectiveness and efficiency and skills, ensuring clinical and corporate governance, evidence-based care supported by evidence-based management, leadership, and use of resources. The best quality of care we can provide from well managed and led staff is our objective, enhancing patient care and the patient experience.

The healthcare environment nationally and internationally is dramatically changing, the pattern of demand is changing, and the technology of medicine, funding, organisation, and structure is changing, too; demand is set on a collision course with supply and this is all happening against a background of economic stringency, cost containment, and demographic change.

In general, healthcare services provision remains funded from taxation and are universal being available to everyone free at the point of provision. Patients expect service responsiveness and choice. There is increasing plurality of provision and this is all set against the paradox of the drive both to greater competition and increased collaboration and partnership. This book, *Key Tools and Techniques in Management and Leadership of the Allied Health Professions*, draws together a range of assessment and measurement tools, techniques, top tips, templates, and guidance. For the first time we are including a CD as part of the publication and soon hope to incorporate the suite on to the Internet. All of the assessments are tried and tested, piloted by ourselves and others, and are evidence-based. We include chapters on, for example, benchmarking, assessment of organisational and management structures, management quality, outcome measures, how our services use staff time, and there is guidance on human resource techniques such as Myers-Briggs and 360° appraisal.

We include templates that can be used and adapted in reporting, for example, clinical governance, human resources, activity, and finance. There are guides on report writing, presentations, and avoidance of time wasting.

We have included sections designed to support managers and leaders to ensure that services thrive or at least do not become eroded in the tough world of economic stringency. We have also included chapters focussing on management of change, care pathway design, and learning and teaching styles.

All of these are essential to management and leadership of the healthcare professions. Many of the chapters will help service monitoring and support managers and leaders develop evidence bases for their services. This evidence is essential for business case development, development of new services, retaining effective services, the provision of clinically effective services, and prioritisation, where the less effective can be jettisoned or decreased in favour of new and more effective approaches. Use of the tools and techniques will increase the confidence of managers and leaders when developing services, preventing loss of valuable services, or retaining the status quo. Developing strong, verifiable evidence that stands up to scrutiny by others is vital.

We are privileged to be authors and editors of this book and wholeheartedly thank our contributors who have generously shared their expertise, experience, and knowledge and have put time in to producing chapters. We also thank our publisher—Radcliffe Publishing Ltd—for their support, encouragement, and the confidence they place in us.

Robert Jones and Fiona Jenkins
May 2011

About the authors

Dr. Robert Jones, PhD, MPhil, BA, FCSP, Grad Dip Phys, CHSM, MMACP Head of Therapy Services Directorate, East Sussex Hospitals NHS Trust.

Robert has management and leadership responsibility for all therapy services in one of the largest Trusts in the UK. He leads a large team of therapy and support staff in acute services, primary care, external contracts, and the independent sector.

A physiotherapist by background, he is a former chair and vice president of the Chartered Society of Physiotherapy and registrant member of the HPC.

He was seconded to the Commission for Health Improvement for a year as the AHP consultant/advisor; he has represented AHPs on an NHS information authority project board and other DH working groups. He has recently completed a five-year term as a Governor of Moorfield's Eye Hospital NHS Foundation Trust.

Robert has led a wide range of successful redesign projects and service innovations, including national exemplars. He has published widely on management and leadership, clinical topics, IM&T in Allied Health Professions, and is Honorary Fellow of the University of Brighton and Plymouth University. His PhD is in management and MPhil is in social policy.

Fiona Jenkins, MA (dist), FCSP, Grad Dip Phys, MHSM, NEBS Dip (M), PGCO Executive Director of Therapies and Health Sciences Cardiff, and Vale University Health Board.

Fiona is director of one of the seven local health boards in Wales, a new post taken up in 2010. Her responsibilities extend to the HPC registered staff, both AHPs and healthcare scientists, in a large organisation, including primary, community, secondary, and tertiary care. She is executive lead for a range of services, including the Professional Forum, Stroke services and Director of Therapies and Healthcare Sciences lead for IM&T. Prior to this she was Clinical Director of Therapies in South Devon. Fiona also previously held the post of Trust service redesign lead.

A former council member and vice president of the Chartered Society of Physiotherapy, Fiona has led and been involved with a large number of service-improvement projects, several of which have been award winning. She has extensive experience of care pathway development and service redesign across the health economy. She has also published widely. Fiona holds an MA (Dist.) in management and is currently undertaking research for a PhD in NHS management related to AHP services.

Fiona and Robert collaboratively lecture both nationally and internationally, lead masterclasses and workshops and give presentations on management and leadership topics and service re-design. They undertake AHP service management reviews and are commissioned for research and surveys.

They successfully completed the INSEAD NHS/Leadership Centre Clinical Strategists' programme at the Business School in Fontainebleau Paris and continue to undertake project work with the university. They have both been members of DH working groups for AHP information management and AHP referral to treatment projects.

They have a range of publications including the series of Allied Health Professions Essential Guides. Their website is www.jjconsulting.org.uk.

List of contributors

Margaret Hastings, MBA, (dist), BA, FCSP
Physiotherapy Manager
West Dumbartonshire CHP NHS Greater Glasgow and
Clyde Clinical Information eHealth Lead,
Chair National Clinical Data Development Programme,
NHS Scotland AHP Information Advisor to Scottish Government Health Department.

Simon Loveday and Sheena Loveday, MPhil, MA, BA
Directors K2 Management Development Ltd.
Cheltenham

Dr. Anne Mandy, PhD, MSc, BSc (Hons.), Cert. Ed
Research Student Division Leader
Principal Research Fellow Clinical Research Centre
University of Brighton

Dr. Gail Louw, PhD, MA, MSc, BA
Formerly Principal Lecturer
Institute of Postgraduate Medicine
Brighton and Sussex Medical School

Kay Mohanna, FRCGP, DCH, PGDipMed, Ed, MA
Senior lecturer, Keele University School of Medicine
Director of Postgraduate Medicine

Dr. Elizabeth Cottrell
Academic Clinical Fellow General Practice
University Hospital North Staffordshire NHS FT and Keele University

David Wall, MB, ChB, PGCE, MMEd, PhD, FRCP, FRCGP
Deputy Regional Postgraduate Dean
West Midlands Deanery
Honorary Professor of Medical Education, Staffordshire University

Ruth Chambers
GP and Honorary Professor Primary Care, Staffordshire University

List of abbreviations

A&E	Accident and Emergency
AHP	Allied Health Profession
BAU	Business as Usual
BPPF	Best Practice Performance Frontier
BPM	Business Performance Management
CABG	Coronary Artery Bypass Graft
CEO	Chief Executive Officer
CHI	Commission for Health Improvement
CIP	Cost Improvement Programmes
CQC	Care Quality Commission
CRES	Cash-Releasing Efficiency Savings
DEA	Data Envelopment Analysis
DH	Department of Health
DNAs	Did Not Attends
DRG	Diagnostic-Related Groups
EBITDA	Earnings Before Interest, Taxes, Depreciation, and Amortisation
ECDL	European Computer Driving Licence
EPR	Electronic Patient Record
FT	Foundation Trust
GDP	Gross Domestic Product
GP	General Practitioner
HIS	Hospital Information Systems
HPC	Health Professions Council

HR	Human Resources
HRG	Healthcare Resource Groups
ICD	International Classification of Disease
ICD-10	International Classifications of Diseases 10th Revision
ICF	International Classification of Functioning, Disability, and Health
ICP	Integrated Care Pathway
ICT	Information and Computer Technologies
IEA	Industrial Excellence Award
IHTSDO	International Health Terminology Standards Development Organisation
IM	Information Management
IM&T	Information Management and Technology
IP	Internet Protocol
IT	Information Technology
KPI	Key Performance Indicator
MBTI	Myers-Briggs Type Indicator
MFF	Market Forces Factor
MOH	Ministry of Health
MQM	Management Quality Matrix
NeLH	National Electronic Library for Health
NHS	National Health Service
NHSI	National Health Service Institute for Innovation and Improvement
NICE	National Institute for Health and Clinical Excellence
NLH	National Library for Health
NLOP	National Local Ownership Programme
NPfIT	National Programme for Information Technology
NPSA	National Patient Safety Agency
OH	Occupational Health
OPCS	Office of Population Censuses and Surveys
PACS	Picture Archiving and Communication System
PAS	Patient Administration System
PBC	Practice-Based Commissioning
PbR	Payment by Results
PC	Personal Computer

PCT	Primary Care Trust
PDA	Personal Digital Assistants
PEST	Political, Economic, Social, Technological
PFI	Private Finance Initiative
PI	Performance Indicator
PR	Public Relations
PROMs	Patient-Reported Outcome Measures
PROMIS	Patient-Reported Outcome Measurement Information System
R&D	Research and Development
RBAC	Role-Based Access Control
RFID	Radio-Frequency Identification
RSS	Really Simple Syndication
RTT	Referral to Treatment Time
SETS	Staffordshire Evaluation of Teaching Styles
SFIs	Standing Financial Instructions
SHA	Strategic Health Authority
SLA	Service-Level Agreement
SLR	Service-Line Reporting
SNFs	Skilled Nurse Facilities
SMART	Specific, Measurable, Achievable, Realistic, Timed
SNOMED	Systematised Nomenclature of Medicine
SSDL	Staged Self-Directed Learning
SUS	Secondary User Service
SWOT	Strength, Weakness, Opportunity, Threat
TCP	Transmission Control Protocol
TQM	Total Quality Management
TUC	Trades Union Congress
UK	United Kingdom
UPI	Unique Patient Identifier
USB	Universal Serial Bus
VAS	Visual Analogue Scale
WHO	World Health Organization
www	World Wide Web

List of templates

Template 17.1: AHP Clinical governance reporting
Template 17.2: AHP services human resources reports
Template 17.3: Example AHP activity report

List of books in the series

Managing and Leading in the Allied Health Professions
Developing the Allied Health Professional
Key Topics in Healthcare Management—understanding the big picture
Managing Money, Measurement and Marketing in the Allied Health Professions
Key Tools and Techniques in Management and Leadership of the Allied Health Professions

CHAPTER 1

Allied Health Professions' Management Quality Matrix

Fiona Jenkins and Robert Jones

INTRODUCTION

If quality and excellence are to be at the heart of service provision and the goals that AHP managers strive to achieve for their services, it is essential to be able to measure performance. In order to determine whether we are achieving management quality, it is necessary to establish whether there is alignment between performance, strategy, vision, and desired outcomes.

In this chapter, we set out our Management Quality Matrix (MQM), which we have designed for the purpose of evaluating a wide range of performance parameters. The Matrix was developed in the context of management quality and strategy drawing on a range of concepts such as performance management, 'Lean', Six Sigma, balanced scorecard, 'dashboards', TQM, and benefits realisation. We recommend that the use of IM&T is integral to accurate, timely, and relevant measurement for Matrix components, although the evaluation can also be undertaken with paper-based information. Measurement is essential to enable meaningful evaluation to take place. We also draw on the management quality, industrial, and healthcare excellence work developed at INSEAD.[1, 2, 3] Also incorporated within the design of the Matrix are ideas from the work of contributors to this series[4, 5, 6] together with our own accumulated knowledge, experience, and research over many years.

The Matrix, which is set out later in this chapter, comprises 14 standards, each incorporating several components broadly reflecting the six dimensions of management quality:

1 communication
2 participation
3 employee development
4 measurement

5   delegation
6   integration

The Matrix will enable AHP managers not simply to engage in 'box ticking' exercises, but rather to measure using metrics indicative of progress toward value and responsiveness for patients. The evaluation facilitates best possible clinical outcomes, efficiency, effectiveness, and optimal resource use whilst acknowledging and using national targets, but not merely being subservient to these. Targets are not goals in themselves; value for the patient is the goal. An important objective of using the Matrix is the improvement of performance in all fields of activity within service management; it will enable managers to identify the need to design and implement processes and initiate effective change. The evaluation can be used for performance management as a useful measure to ensure understanding of true performance and as a comparison through time for continuous improvement as well as internal benchmarking. As an external benchmarking process, it can be used to draw performance comparisons between provider organisations. It may also be used for supporting the management process as an ad hoc service review tool and might also be useful to use in conjunction with our Service Review Assessment of AHP management structures.[4]

Developing strategy and measuring performance requires participation at all levels. For the achievement of success, actions or activities need to be aligned. It may be helpful to ask ourselves a number of key questions:
• is everyone in the team 'pulling' in the same direction?
• does the direction benefit the patient?
• are there baseline measures?
• are we measuring so that we know whether we are improving or not?
• do staff have the training and motivation to provide value and bring about improvement?
• are tensions around fear of change recognised and managed?
• are problems/mistakes treated as opportunities to improve?

Our Matrix is not only an annual measurement assessment; it can be used to support management quality development throughout the year, assessing progress in strategy and operational developments.

It is not our purpose here to discuss management theories in detail, but an overview of some key definitions and concepts are outlined in order to place the Matrix in context.

METRICS

The term 'metrics' relates to standards of measurement through which efficiency, performance, progress, quality of a process, plan, or product is assessed. Examples of these measures, or 'metrics', include indicators, targets, and benchmarks of performance.

KEY PERFORMANCE INDICATORS (KPIs)

A KPI is a tool for service improvement, focusing upon significant measurements that indicate degree of success or lack of achievement. A KPI is a composite of:
* a measure of the performance against specific goals or objectives
* a target (or targets)
* an action resulting from the measurement.

BUSINESS PERFORMANCE MANAGEMENT (BPM)

BPM consists of a set of management and analytical processes supported by IM&T and paper systems that enables services to define strategic goals and then measure and manage performance. Core BPM processes include, for example, clinical activity and financial performance; operational planning; reporting; modelling; monitoring of key performance indicators; clinical governance; and human resources. BPM involves consolidation of data from various sources, analysis of the data, and putting the learning into practice. It enhances processes by creating better feedback loops and can help to identify and eliminate problems.

LEAN THINKING

'Lean' was developed by Toyota, becoming integral to its industrial engineering processes. The overall objective is to eliminate non-value-added waste to reduce process cycle times, improve delivery performance, and reduce costs. This approach is adopted with the objective of improving flow; it is about getting the right things to the right places at the right time, in the right quantities.[7] In the context of healthcare, 'Lean' facilitates patient-focused service provision and is intended to help the patient through adding value. It is designed to eliminate the root causes of non-value-added activities such as patients waiting between activities during care.

In eliminating waste, quality improves and at the same time, overall activity time decreases and consequently costs decrease. A further objective is to improve patient flow or 'smoothness' of work, eliminating unevenness in the pathway, not only waste.

Lean brings into many industries, including healthcare, new concepts, tools, and methods that have been effectively utilised to improve process flow. Tools that address workplace organisation, standardisation, visual control, and elimination of non-value-added steps are applied to improve flow, eliminate waste, and exceed patient expectation.[8]

In order to eliminate waste and ensure evenness of process, the phases or steps in it must be examined to make the process visible so that waste or unevenness is highlighted and can be rectified. Questions might include those in Box 1.1.

> **Box 1.1** Questions to ask to eliminate waste
> 1   Are the steps within the process clear or are parts difficult to identify?
> 2   Are responsibilities clear for each individual and for teams?
> 3   Who carries overall responsibility for the entire process?
> 4   Are there unnecessary phases in the process?
> 5   Are the right facilities or consumables available when required?
> 6   Are the processes 'joined-up'?
> 7   Are the measures and targets appropriate and relevant to the process?
> 8   Do problems continually recur and need 'fixing' or is appropriate time taken
>   out to 'fix' the system once and for all?
> 9   Are there gaps, duplications, or bottlenecks in the service?

It may be useful to adopt the well-tested management technique of 'five whys'—asking 'why' five times as in root cause analysis.[9]

The following example demonstrates the basic process.

Patients have long waits for treatment (the problem).

1   *Why?* Not enough treatment slots available (first why).
2   *Why?* Mismatch between new and follow-up appointment slots (second why).
3   *Why?* Capacity and demand has not been modelled (third why).
4   *Why?* Booking process not fully understood or process mapped (fourth why).
5   *Why?* Lacking service improvement and innovative skills in the service (fifth why, a root cause).

The NHSI Productive Series[10] supports NHS teams to redesign and streamline the way they manage and work. This aims to achieve significant and lasting improvements predominately in the extra time that they give to patients, as well as improving the quality of care delivered whilst reducing costs.

In a recent survey undertaken by NHSI,[10] significant areas of time wasting in management were identified, for example:

- on average, leaders spend only 7.5% of time on planning, reflecting, and thinking
- of the average 54-hour week worked by an NHS manager, 38 hours were spent in meetings
- of the 26 meetings attended, only seven started on time
- only 36% of attendees actively participated in the meetings.

SIX SIGMA

The fundamental purpose of Six Sigma is the implementation of a measurement-based strategy that focuses on process improvement and variation reduction. The technique was developed for quality engineering using statistical techniques to facilitate understanding and measure and reduce process variation with the goal of improving service quality and cost. The methodology adopts the use of structured techniques to reduce defects. Technically, Six Sigma is a disciplined, data-driven approach and methodology for eliminating defects '(driving toward six standard deviations between the mean and the nearest specification limit) in any process'.[11] The word 'sigma' is a statistical term that measures how far a particular process deviates from perfection. A crucial idea behind Six Sigma is that the number of defects in a process is measured in order that they can be eliminated in a systematic way aiming to be as close as possible to 'zero defects' in the process.

The concept of Six Sigma is applicable in healthcare. The DMAIC process (define, measure, analyse, improve, and control)—which is consistent with evidence-based healthcare practice—is an improvement system[11] for existing processes falling below specification and looking for incremental improvement.

Box 1.2 Six Sigma DMAIC process
- *Define*: process improvement goals that are consistent with patient requirements and the enterprise strategy.
- *Measure*: key aspects of the current process and collect relevant data.
- *Analyse*: the data to verify cause-and-effect relationships; determine what the relationships are and attempt to ensure that all factors have been considered.
- *Improve*: or optimise the process based on data analysis.
- *Control*: to ensure that any deviations from target are corrected before they result in defects; set up pilot runs to establish process capability, set up control mechanisms, and continually monitor the process.

On the other hand, the Six Sigma DMADV (define, measure, analyse, design, and verify) process is an improvement system used to develop new processes, services, or pathways, for example.

TOTAL QUALITY MANAGEMENT

TQM, a Japanese-inspired concept, is an approach centred on improved organisational performance and effectiveness. Deming[12, 13] emphasised the importance of visionary leadership and the responsibility of senior management for initiating change. One of Deming's 14 principles was to eliminate slogans as he argued the importance of doing the right things the first time. He focused on the importance of good management, including the human side of quality improvement and how employees should be treated. This is an approach centred on quality, based on the participation of an organisation's staff, and aiming at long-term success. The 'total' in TQM applies to the organisation or service as a whole; it also applies to all of the activities, including culture, ethics, and attitude.

TQM is far wider in its application than just assuring product or service quality—it is a way of managing people and business processes to ensure complete customer satisfaction at every stage, internally and externally. TQM, combined with effective leadership, results in an organisation doing the right things right the first time.[14]

Pentecost[15] identified key elements of TQM that can be adapted for healthcare services as shown in Box 1.3.

Box 1.3 Key elements of TQM

1 A total process—involving all management units in the organisation, and led from the top.
2 The patient is 'king' with every strategy, process, and action directly related to satisfying customers' needs.
3 A greater emphasis on rational information collection and analysis.
4 Emphasis on a different approach to looking at the costs of poor quality by examining all processes that add to costs.
5 A greater involvement of staff, recognising that they are a great untapped resource.
6 Teamwork—involving multidisciplinary and multilevel working in problem solving and to meet patients' needs.
7 The requirements of creative thinking and the ability to think beyond the immediate job or working environment.

Other authors add leadership as a key principle as leaders establish unity of purpose, direction, and the internal environment of the service, creating the environment in which all staff can become involved in achieving the service objectives.

BENEFITS REALISATION

This approach is the identification of target benefits, their definition, planning, structuring, and realisation resulting from investing in change. Projects, service changes, and service redesign are undertaken to deliver benefits for service users. However, the majority of projects and programmes are criticised for failing to achieve the predicted objectives or benefits. There are a number of possible reasons for this, including, for example:
- business cases being focused on financial targets rather than being expressed in terms of the benefits that can be understood and implemented
- too much emphasis on outcomes that on their own do not provide specific benefits
- no mechanisms or structures to manage the realisation of benefits.

It is very important to identify clear benefits that relate to unambiguous service objectives and to assign ownership to the people responsible for ensuring and managing their achievement.

The challenge for organisations is in identifying clear benefits, assigning ownership, determining how they can be measured, and then making sure how they can be delivered. Benefit planning, management, and realisation sets out to bring structure, accountability, and discipline to the delivery of the benefits inherent in projects.[15]

Important aspects of this approach are:

- the way objectives and benefits are expressed and structured
- differentiating between objectives, outcomes, benefits, and also financial results
- the whole planning and management of the process.

CLINICAL DASHBOARD

High-quality information is an important element in the facilitation of good performance among clinical and management teams and helps to promote that the right services and best care are provided. A 'dashboard' is a 'tool set' of visual displays specifically designed to provide relevant and timely information to inform decision-making. Dashboards provide data captured in a visual and useable format. It may display local information alongside the relevant national metrics.

The development of clinical dashboards was a key recommendation for 'The Next Stage Review'.[16]

Box 1.4 Five major features of clinical dashboards[17]

1 Provide better information for clinical teams presented in easy-to-understand formats, with high visual impact.
2 Utilise multiple sources of existing data.
3 Provide information relevant across multidisciplinary teams.
4 Information provided in 'real' time with no delay for data cleansing.
5 Allows configuration to local requirements and comparison against national data sets.

NHS information sets and initiatives are complimented by clinical dashboards by providing locally required indicators configured to local needs, supporting clinical teams to deliver faster, improved, and safer quality of care. Clinical dashboards are widely adapted for management purposes.

BALANCED SCORECARD

Balanced scorecards are strategic planning and management 'tools' used in many types of organisations worldwide, including healthcare, to align business activities to the vision and strategy of the organisation, improve internal and external communications, and monitor organisational performance against strategic goals. The balanced scorecard approach was developed by Kaplan and Norton as a performance measurement framework that added strategic, customer-focused, and learning measures as non-financial performance measures to traditional financial metrics to give managers a more balanced view of organisational performance.[18] The balanced scorecard provides a framework for the provision of performance measurement and supports managers to identify what should be done and measured. This methodology is designed for the purpose of transforming the service strategic plan into action.

Box 1.5 Reasons for implementing the balanced scorecard approach
- Increased focus on strategy and results.
- Measuring what matters to improve performance.
- Align organisational strategy with the work people do day to day.
- Focus on the drivers for future performance.
- Improve communication of the service vision and strategy.
- Prioritise projects and initiatives.

The balanced scorecard suggests that we view the organisation from four perspectives and develop metrics, collect data, and analyse it relative to each of these perspectives.[18]

The four perspectives of balanced scorecards are:
1 learning and growth
2 the business process perspective
3 the service user perspective
4 financial perspective.

In healthcare settings, there is a growing consensus that financial indicators alone are not an adequate measure of performance and that a broader view is needed. The balanced scorecard approach is increasingly used in healthcare organisations as a means of improving performance. The NHS has a very difficult task of fulfiling a wide range of different and complex objectives due to the scope and diversity of the service; the balanced scorecard can be used to support in formal recognition and measurement of objectives.

AHP MANAGEMENT QUALITY MATRIX

Frameworks for strategy must incorporate the vision, objectives, and policies of AHP services setting out the purpose, plans, and actions for implementation. Without explicit strategy, it will be difficult for AHP services to coordinate action and measure performance. To achieve the benefits of 'joined up' working, it is necessary for people to collaborate, and the absence of explicit strategy will result in staff working at cross-purposes. Strategy must be communicated clearly to enable corporate understanding and 'ownership' at all levels. This requires operational activity to be put in place so that performance can be measured and appropriate learning, change, and subsequent action be put in place as necessary.

To succeed, AHP services need structured, strategic frameworks to provide starting points for progress and a means for assessment and evaluation. Our Management Quality Evaluation Matrix is based on AHP strategy and is intended to enable AHP managers to be explicit about their service strategies, facilitating measurement of performance in respect to service provision, activity, processes, people, resources, and systems.

Our Evaluation Matrix is designed to enable AHP managers to measure performance; if performance is not measured, it is not managed. An important objective is to enable managers to work toward improving the overall effectiveness, efficiency, and responsiveness—in short, the overall quality of services. The Evaluation Matrix is used to evaluate performance against standards on a forward-looking basis so that variances are detected and appropriate actions taken. The Matrix incorporates 14 key Standards for managing AHP services, each being subdivided into components that make up specific management quality sections within it.

Box 1.6 The 14 AHP Management Quality Standards
 1 Strategy.
 2 Patient and service user experience.
 3 Clinical excellence.
 4 Finance.
 5 Information and metrics.
 6 Activity.
 7 Staff resource effectiveness.
 8 Staff management and development.
 9 Service improvement and redesign.
10 Leadership and management development.
11 Risk management.
12 Corporate governance.
13 Communications and marketing.
14 Key performance indicators.

The evaluation of each component has been designed to give information that is easy to interpret. A number of methods are used for evaluating components, for example: yes/no, percentage achievement, or requiring data or text. It may be appropriate to include graphs and bar charts in some places. There is space in the Matrix for comments to be recorded. Each Standard requires a summary and action planning by the AHP manager when reviewing the management quality of their service.

The evaluation gives an overview of the strengths and weaknesses of the service and where there may be opportunity for improvement and development. When completed, it will also contain valuable data on activity and financial performance.

The Matrix can be used for unidisciplinary AHP services or multiple services where these are managed collectively. When assessing multiple AHP services, each profession **should be evaluated separately**.

An important objective of the evaluation is to give guidance and to help focus attention on the service. It is not intended that each and every strategy and component be fully achieved at first, although some managers may be successful in the majority of components within each Standard. It may be helpful to focus on one Standard at a time, gradually developing the Matrix over a period.

In this way, the Matrix can be used to guide management quality development in AHP services. The Matrix can also be used as an aid to the management process as a prompt to instigating work and projects on management quality throughout the service and as an easy source for information retrieval to be used on an ongoing basis.

Standard 1 strategy

The service has a documented strategy that is reviewed and updated annually.

Component	Evaluation		Comment
1.1 Organisational strategy; does your organisation have a strategy?	YES	NO	
1.2 Do you have an up-to-date strategy for your service that is currently available? • Is this aligned to the organisational strategy?	YES	NO	
1.3 Is there a 'value statement' that is shared by staff in your service? • If yes, please detail.	YES	NO	
1.4 Service mission statement/vision; is this agreed and documented and up to date? • If yes, please detail.	YES	NO	
1.5 Service portfolio—the range of services you provide and have responsibility for; is this documented? • What service specifications do you have? Please list.	YES	NO	

Component	Evaluation		Comment
1.6 Major goals/objectives for your service; are these documented? • What are they? Please list.	YES	NO	
1.7 Which service level strategies do you currently have? • Financial savings? • Education and training? • Information management and technology? • Marketing? • Clinical governance? • Patient and public involvement? • Quality? • Service improvement?	YES	NO	
1.8 Do you have organisational charts for your service illustrating your structure, governance, and management team? • please attach	YES	NO	
1.9 Do you produce a service annual report outlining, for example: • Key achievements against, e.g. target, benchmarks? • Aspirations for continuing service improvement/ development? • Activity analysis? • Finance report? • Key performance indicators and performance? • Quality? • Human resource report? • Marketing strategy? • Clinical governance report?	YES	NO	
Standard summary and action:			

Standard 2 patient and service user experience

Patients' views and experiences are actively sought and incorporated into service redesign.

Component	Evaluation		Comment
2.1 Does your service use patient survey data to benchmark its services to patients? • If yes, can you provide evidence where you have used this to improve services?	YES	NO	

Component	Evaluation		Comment
2.2 Do you actively encourage views from patients about services provided: • How is this done, e.g. surveys, focus groups?	YES	NO	
2.3 Are compliments monitored within your service and action plans put in place as appropriate? • Detail how learning is disseminated.	YES	NO	
2.4 Are complaints monitored within your service? • Detail any action plans put in place.	YES	NO	
2.5 Do all staff collect patient outcome data? • What outcomes and measures are used?		%	
2.6 Is patient outcome data analysed?		%	
2.7 Do you have a procedure for offering patient chaperones?	YES	NO	
2.8 Do you actively involve patients in informed decision-making about their care? • How do you monitor this?	YES	NO	
2.9 Do you have agreed, evidence-based protocols and pathways in use? • If yes, please detail.	YES	NO	
2.10 Is there a mechanism in place to ensure compliance with NICE (National Institute for Health and Clinical Excellence) guidelines?	YES	NO	
2.11 Do you undertake environment audits in patient treatment areas?	YES	NO	
2.12 Does your service have a quality-monitoring programme for the production and review of patient information leaflets? • List the leaflets you have updated in the last year.	YES	NO	
2.13 Do you have a website that the public can access information about your services?	YES	NO	
2.14 Do you monitor waiting times and put action plans in place as necessary?	YES	NO	
Standard summary and action:			

Standard 3 clinical excellence

The service demonstrates procedures and practices to ensure high-quality patient care.

Component	Evaluation		Comment
3.1 Does your service have representation on the organisation's: • Senior clinicians committee? • Clinical governance committee? • Audit committee? • Research and development committee?	YES	NO	
3.2 Are there regular clinical governance review meetings within your service and appropriate action plans put in place?	YES	NO	
3.3 Are there arrangements in place for clinical audits? • Please list audits reported in the last year.	YES	NO	
3.4 Is the requirement to undertake clinical audit included in staff job descriptions?	YES	NO	
3.5 Is there a mechanism for reporting results and implementing the recommendations from clinical audits?	YES	NO	
3.6 Do you have staff undertaking research and development projects? • If so, list current projects.	1. 2. 3. 4. 5.		
3.7 Do you have mechanisms to ensure the provision of evidence-based practice, for example: • Staff appraisal and personal development plans • In-service education and training • Access to continued professional development • Peer review • Staff access to the Internet • Staff access to library facilities/journals • Journal review sessions • Participation in professional networks • Active links with higher education institutions • Staff undertaking higher degrees • Clinicals supervision • Mentoring	YES	NO	
3.8 Is there a staff education and training policy in place?	YES	NO	
3.9 Do you have standards for clinical record keeping?	YES	NO	
3.10 Are your clinical records monitored regularly against a set standard?	YES	NO	

Component	Evaluation		Comment
3.11 Do you have procedures in place for obtaining and recording informed patient consent?	YES	NO	
3.12 Do you have mechanisms in place for obtaining patient feedback on service quality? • If yes, please detail.	YES	NO	
3.13 Are lessons learned from feedback incorporated into practice? • What is the evidence?	YES	NO	
3.14 Has your service established procedures for developing and implementing? • Clinical guidelines • NICE guidelines • Care pathways	YES	NO	
3.15 Do you provide services that contribute to the public health agenda, regarding self-management and prevention? Such as: • Obesity management • Healthy lifestyles/exercise	YES	NO	
3.16 Have you developed staff with extended scope skills? Such as: supplementary prescribing, injection therapy, and radiographic interpretation • Please detail.	YES	NO	
Standard summary:	**Action:**		

Standard 4 finance

There is comprehensive monitoring and knowledge of the service finances within your management teams and the service is financially viable.

Component	Evaluation		Comment
4.1 Are you the budget holder for your service and responsible for budget management?	YES	NO	
4.2 Do you have monthly budget statements that you analyse?	YES	NO	
4.3 Do you monitor your financial performance on at least a monthly basis? • What monitoring method do you use?	YES	NO	

Component	Evaluation		Comment
4.4 Do you have controls in place regarding authorisation of purchases?	YES	NO	
4.5 What is your annual budget? • Pay • Non-pay • Income			
4.6 Overspend/underspend position last financial year?			
4.7 Reasons for over/underspend?			
4.8 Do you have income-generation projects? • If yes, please detail.	YES	NO	
4.9 What type of contracts do you have? For example: • Block contract? • Cost per case? • Cost per contact? • Cost and volume?			
4.10 Do you have any service-level agreements? • If yes, what is your income from service-level agreements?			
4.11 Do you have any external contracts? • If yes, what is your annual profit from external contracts?			
4.12 Do you have contacts with voluntary organisations? • If yes, what is your annual income from voluntary organisations?			
4.13 What is your annual income from hiring out facilities/equipment?			
4.14 Do you have income identified from payment by results?			
4.15 Are your service costs identifiable by service-line reporting?	YES	NO	
4.16 Do you know what your reference costs are? • If yes, how do these relate to the national picture?			
4.17 What are your earnings before interest, taxes, depreciation, and amortisation (EBITDA)?			
4.18 Do you have an inventory of equipment for your service documented?			
4.19 Do you have stock-control programmes in place?			

Component	Evaluation	Comment
4.20 Are you required to implement cost-improvement programmes and cash-releasing efficiency savings? • What percentage target do you have this year? • What programmes do you have in place for meeting it?		
4.21 Does your service have charitable trust funds with monitoring in place?		
Standard summary:	**Action:**	

Standard 5 information and metrics

The service gathers timely, accurate, and relevant data as a by-product of clinical activity. Appropriate metrics are used for clinical and managerial purposes.

Component	Evaluation		Comment
5.1 Does your service have a data collection system that is fit for purpose?	YES	NO	
5.2 Does your service have a computerised data-collection system fit for purpose?	YES	NO	
5.3 Do clinicians input data at the same time that treatment takes place (real time)?	YES	NO	
5.4 Is your information system capable of providing accurate, timely, and relevant reports?	YES	NO	
5.5 Are you able to report referral to treatment time for all referrals received?	YES	NO	
5.6 Do you collect and use data for clinical audits?	YES	NO	
5.7 Do you collect and use data for staff activity analysis?	YES	NO	
5.8 Do you collect and use data for staff case load analysis?	YES	NO	
5.9 Do you collect and analyse patient outcome data for all patients?	%		
5.10 Where there are gaps in metrics, are you developing ways to measure the quality of services? • Please detail gaps.	YES	NO	
5.11 Do your clinical staff input the data themselves?	YES	NO	

Component	Evaluation		Comment
5.12 Do your clerical staff input data? Are there gaps or duplication in the data?	YES	NO	
5.13 Do you have an agreed and current protocol for data sharing?	YES	NO	
Standard summary:	**Action:**		

Standard 6 activity

Activity is reviewed and analysed on a monthly and annual basis for performance management and for projections for the coming year.

Component	Sub-component	Total		Comment
6.1 All staff record activity data on the same day that the activity is performed.		YES	NO	
6.2 Total service throughput last financial year, defined by total referrals, new patients, and total attendances?	Total referrals			
	New patients			
	Total attendances			
6.3 What was your new to follow-up ratio last financial year for each service? (Name each service.)	1.	1:		
	2.	1:		
	3.	1:		
	4.	1:		
	5.	1:		
6.4 Do you analyse your re-referral rate and use this for service planning?		YES	NO	
6.5 What is your anticipated (planned) total service throughput for the next financial year?	New patients			
	Total attendances			
6.6 What are your out patient referral to treatment times for each service? (Name each service.)	1.		weeks	
	2.		weeks	
	3.		weeks	
	4.		weeks	
	5.		weeks	

Component	Sub-component	Total		Comment
6.7 Are you able to report RTT (referral to treatment time) for all patients referred?		YES	NO	
6.8 What are your service DNA (did not attend) percentage rates? (Name each service.)	1.		%	
	2.		%	
	3.		%	
	4.		%	
	5.		%	
6.9 Do you have a demand and capacity management plan in place? • If yes, please detail.		YES	NO	
6.10 Do you analyse your staff activity time to review the time allocation between patient contact time, patient-related activity, and non-patient-related activity?		YES	NO	
6.11 What is your service standard response time for inpatient service provision? (Name each service.)	1.		days	
	2.		days	
	3.		days	
	4.		days	
	5.		days	
6.12 Illustrate your referral trend to your whole service during last five years. • (Insert a graph/bar chart with this information.)				
6.13 Illustrate your capacity plan projection for next year. • (Insert a graph/bar chart with this information.)				
6.14 Illustrate your did not attend trend to your whole service during last five years. • (Insert a graph/bar chart with this information.)				
Standard summary and action:				

Standard 7 staff resources

There is a comprehensive knowledge and understanding of the staff resources used by the service and they are deployed effectively and reviewed frequently.

Component	Evaluation	Comment
7.1 What is the head count of your AHP staff group?		
7.2 What is the whole time equivalent grade profile of each of your AHP staff groups: • Band 2 • Band 3 • Band 4 • Band 5 • Band 6 • Band 7 • Band 8a • Band 8b • Band 8c • Band 8d • Band 9 • Director	WTE WTE WTE WTE WTE WTE WTE WTE WTE WTE WTE WTE	
7.3 What is your ratio of registered to non-registered staff	:	
7.4 What is your service annual staff turnover?	%	
7.5 How do your turnover figures compare with the:		
• National average for your service?	+/- %	
• Your organisation average? (You may wish to include a graph.)	+/- %	
7.6 What is your annual percentage absence through: • Sickness • Maternity leave • Study leave • Other authorised paid leave • Unpaid leave	 % % % % %	
How does this compare with your organisation as a whole?	+/- %	
• Sickness • Maternity leave • Study leave • Other authorised paid leave • Unpaid leave	% % % % %	
7.7 Staff Activity—what is the aggregate percentage staff time spent on: • Patient-related activity • Non-patient-related activity	 % %	

Component	Evaluation		Comment
7.8 Does the service have sufficient expertise to provide comprehensive in-service education/ training? • If yes, please detail.	YES	NO	
7.9 Does the service undertake succession planning?	YES	NO	
7.10 Does every member of staff have an up-to-date job description and knowledge and skills framework (KSF)?	YES	NO	
Standard summary:	**Action:**		

Standard 8 staff management, education, and development

Staff are managed, supported, and developed to meet clinical, organisational, and professional requirements.

Component	Evaluation		Comment
8.1 Have you benchmarked your staffing establishment against similar organisations?	YES	NO	
8.2 If you have benchmarked how do you compare? • Please detail.			
8.3 What is the ratio between HPC-registered AHP staff to assistants?	:		
8.4 What is the ratio between HPC-registered AHP staff to clerical staffing?	:		
8.5 What is your service percentage compliance with mandatory training attendance requirements?	%		
8.6 What is your service percentage compliance for undertaking annual development reviews (appraisal)?	%		
8.7 Is your staff HPC registration checked annually for compliance?	YES	NO	
8.8 Are the numbers of staff grievances/disciplinary investigations monitored on an ongoing basis?	YES	NO	

Component	Evaluation		Comment
8.9 Is there a monitoring procedure in place for staff competence?	YES	NO	
8.10 Is there a staff education and training policy in place?	YES	NO	
8.11 Is a record of all staff training and education kept and regularly updated?	YES	NO	
8.12 Is there a mechanism in place for clinical supervision? • If yes, please detail.	YES	NO	
8.13 Do you have a mentorship or coaching scheme in place? • If yes, please detail.	YES	NO	
8.14 Does your service have clinical specialists?	YES	NO	
8.15 Does your service have extended scope practitioners/advanced practitioners?	YES	NO	
8.16 Does your service have consultant AHP posts?	YES	NO	
8.17 Do you have a study leave policy?	YES	NO	
8.18 Does the service take AHP students? • If there are established links with the higher education institution(s) please detail.	YES	NO	
Standard summary:	**Action:**		

Standard 9 service improvement and redesign

The service actively undertakes redesign and service improvement.

Component	Evaluation		Comment
9.1 Does your service have representation on your organisation's strategic service improvement group or equivalent?	YES	NO	
9.2 Is service improvement embedded in staff job descriptions?	YES	NO	

Component	Evaluation		Comment
9.3 Has your service undertaken redesign projects in the last financial year? List: 1. 2. 3. 4. 5.	YES	NO	
9.4 Does your service have redesign projects in progress during the current financial year? List: 1. 2. 3. 4. 5.	YES	NO	
9.5 Is your service involved in multidisciplinary service improvement projects? List: 1. 2 3 4 5	YES	NO	
9.6 Have you undertaken 'horizon scanning' of other services (internal/external) to inform your service improvement needs?	YES	NO	
9.7 Has your service been recognised at local or national level for innovative service improvement? • If yes, please detail.	YES	NO	
9.8 Are all levels of staff involved in the service redesign initiatives?	YES	NO	
9.9 Do you have user involvement in service redesign? • If yes, please detail.	YES	NO	
9.10 Do you evaluate service improvement initiatives as part of a continuous cycle of improvement?	YES	NO	
9.11 Do you have staff trained with service improvement techniques to undertake service redesign? • If yes please detail.	YES	NO	

Component	Evaluation		Comment
9.12 Do you have staff trained with project management skills?	YES	NO	
Standard summary:	**Action:**		

Standard 10 leadership and management development

The service has effective leadership and management arrangements in place at all levels.

Component	Evaluation		Comment
10.1 Does the organisational structure support effective leadership and management?	YES	NO	
10.2 Does the structure have clearly defined levels of accountability, authority, and delegation?			
10.3 Is leadership and management development included in personal development plans?	YES	NO	
10.4 Is there a leadership/management development programme in place for your staff?	YES	NO	
10.5 What percentage of staff in leadership/ management positions has undertaken this training?		%	
10.6 Does your service have access to leadership development programmes at: • Local level? • National level? • International level?	YES	NO	
10.7 Can you identify projects within or on behalf of your organisation that your service had led during the last year? (List.)	1.		
	2.		
	3.		
	4.		
	5.		
10.8 Have you identified projects within your organisation that your service will be leading during the next year? (List.)	1.		
	2.		
	3.		
	4.		
	5.		

Component	Evaluation		Comment
10.9 Do you have staff members involved in work at national level with professional bodies/regulators?	YES	NO	
10.10 What percentage of staff in management positions has undertaken management training?		%	
10.11 Are you responsible and accountable for performance management of your service?	YES	NO	
10.12 Are you a member of, or represented on, the management committees/boards within your organisation? • If yes, please list.	YES	NO	
10.13 Do you have networks at: • National level? • International level?	YES	NO	
Standard summary:	**Action:**		

Standard 11 risk management

Risk is measured, evaluated, and managed effectively with action plans put in place.

Component	Evaluation		Comment
11.1 Does your service maintain an ongoing, up-to-date risk register, including action logs?	YES	NO	
11.2 Does your service risk register input to the organisation's risk register?	YES	NO	
11.3 Does your service undertake equality impact assessments and comply with standards?	YES	NO	
11.4 Does your service maintain an ongoing, up-to-date register of serious untoward incidents and 'near misses' with action plans in place?	YES	NO	
11.5 Is your service included in the organisation's major incident planning?	YES	NO	
11.6 Does your service undertake litigation audits and have action plans?	YES	NO	
11.7 Is there a mechanism in place for ensuring that national patient safety alerts are communicated throughout the teams and action plans put in place?	YES	NO	

Component	Evaluation		Comment
11.8 Are legal claims monitored and reviewed within your service?	YES	NO	
11.9 Is there a named lead for risk management for each location within your service?	YES	NO	
11.10 Are health and safety assessments undertaken on an ongoing basis?	YES	NO	
11.11 Does your service have a named fire officer?	YES	NO	
11.12 Is staff attendance at mandatory training monitored?	YES	NO	
11.13 Is training in risk management undertaken by your staff?	YES	NO	
Standard summary:	**Action:**		

Standard 12 corporate governance

The service is compliant with the rules, processes, and laws within which your organisation is required to operate and is regulated.

Component	Evaluation		Comment
12.1 Are you aware of and compliant with the 'Nolan' principles of conduct in public life?	YES	NO	
12.2 Have you read and signed your concordance with the organisation's standing financial instructions?	YES	NO	
12.3 Does your service have an identifiable line of reporting to the organisation's board?	YES	NO	
12.4 Do all staff have signed contracts of employment at the time of taking up employment?	YES	NO	
12.5 Do all staff have up-to-date job descriptions?	YES	NO	
12.6 Do all staff members in your service have clearly defined lines of accountability?	YES	NO	
12.7 Do you have a mechanism for recording declarations of interest?	YES	NO	
12.8 Do you have a mechanism in place to ensure that staff comply with professional regulation requirements (HPC)?	YES	NO	
12.9 Do you have a monitoring system in place for checking registration status of all your staff?	YES	NO	

Component	Evaluation		Comment
12.10 Do you have a list of authorised signatories for your service? For example: • Time sheets • Travel claims • Equipment and supplies ordering • Charitable trust funds • Petty cash	YES	NO	
Standard summary:	**Action:**		

Standard 13 communication and marketing

The service has effective internal and external communication processes and well-developed links to ensure service marketing.

Component	Evaluation		Comment
13.1 Is there a communication mechanism within your service to keep staff informed and gather views from staff? • Please detail methods.	YES	NO	
13.2 Have you undertaken a SWOT analysis for your services and developed an action plan? • If yes, please attach.	YES	NO	
13.3 Have you undertaken a PEST analysis for your service and developed an action plan? • If yes, please attach.	YES	NO	
13.4 Do you have an overview of the population served by your service?	YES	NO	
13.5 Is a summary of the 'target' population(s) (market segment) for your service documented?	YES	NO	
13.6 Have you developed service specification(s) for your service?	YES	NO	
13.7 Do you have a Web site for your service? Including, for example: • Locations • Opening times • Facilities • Key managers' contact details • How to contact the service • Referral to service • Service exclusions • Patient information leaflets	YES	NO	

Component	Evaluation		Comment
• Self referral information • Key policies • Expertise available			
13.8 Do you meet multicultural requirements in the form of: • Leaflets in different languages? • Leaflets in different media, e.g. large print? • Access to interpreters? • Access to signers for deaf people?	YES	NO	
13.9 Have you developed links with local media to inform the public about your service?	YES	NO	
13.10 Do you have links and have you developed information about your service for voluntary organisations?	YES	NO	
13.11 Specify the resources that give your service a competitive advantage: • Core competencies • Key assets • Core or critical processes such as pathways	Please detail:		
13.12 What are the major types of uncertainty: • Uncertain demand? • Uncertain staff availability? • Uncertainty of funding streams? • Competitor actions? • Technology/treatment changes?	Please detail:		
13.13 Have you undertaken an analysis of predicted changes in population and made an assessment of possible future demand?	YES	NO	
13.14 Have you established what future commissioner/planning intentions are?	YES	NO	
13.15 Have you established projected future demand from within your own organisation?	YES	NO	
13.16 Are mechanisms in place for teams to communicate across functional boundaries? • If yes, please detail.	YES	NO	
13.17 Have you developed business cases for service developments, improvements, and redesign in light of your market assessment and other relevant factors? • If yes please detail.	YES	NO	
Standard summary:	**Action:**		

Standard 14 top five key performance indicators

The service has identified five top KPIs and monitors progress against them annually.

NB. The KPIs selected will depend upon the service and the strategic priorities. They will therefore vary from service to service and change over time. Identify the top five indicators rating performance.

Component	Evaluation	Comment
14.1		
14.2		
14.3		
14.4		
14.5		
Standard summary:		**Action:**

Management Quality overall action plan		
The following template is designed to copy and paste in the actions identified. This will enable you to monitor them collectively.		
Standard number	Standard action	Review date
1		
2		
3		
4		
5		
6		
7		
8		
9		
10		
11		
12		
13		
14		

Management Quality record of Standard completion and review dates			
Year: 20__	Service:		
Standard	*Date completed*	*Review date*	*Sign-off manager name*
1 Strategy			
2 Patient and service user experience			
3 Clinical excellence			
4 Finance			
5 Information and metrics			
6 Activity			
7 Staff resource effectiveness			
8 Staff management and development			
9 Service improvement and redesign			
10 Leadership and management development			
11 Risk management			
12 Corporate governance			
13 Communications and marketing			
14 Key performance indicators			

REFERENCES

1. Chick S, Huchzermeier C, Loch C. Management quality and operational excellence. In: Jones R, Jenkins F, editors. *Managing Money, Measurement and Marketing for the Allied Health Professions*. Oxford: Radcliffe Publishing; 2010.
2. Loch C, Van der Heyden L, Van Wassenhove L, *et al. Industrial Excellence*. Berlin: Springer; 2003.
3. Loch C, Chick S, Huchzermeier A. *Industrial Excellence Award, Healthcare Questionnaire*. Fontainebleau, INSEAD; 2009.
4. Jones R, Jenkins F. *Managing and Leading in the Allied Health Professions*. Oxford: Radcliffe Publishing; 2006.
5. Jones R, Jenkins F. *Developing the Allied Health Professional*. Oxford: Radcliffe Publishing; 2006.
6. Jones R, Jenkins F. *Key Topics in Healthcare Management—understanding the big picture*. Oxford: Radcliffe Publishing; 2006.
7. Womack J, Jones D. *Lean Thinking: banish waste and create wealth in your corporation, revised and updated*. London: Simon and Schuster; 2003.
8. NHS Institute for Innovation and Improvement. *The Lean Simulation Suitcase*. 2009; www.institute.nhs.uk.

9. Latino R, Latino K. *Root Cause Analysis: improving performance for bottom line results.* Boca Raton, FL: Taylor and Francis; 2006.
10. Six Sigma. 2009; www.isixsigma.com.
11. Deming WE. *Out of the Crisis.* Cambridge, MA: MIT; 1986.
12. Deming WE. *The New Economics for Industry.* Cambridge, MA: MIT; 1993.
13. Department for Business Innovation and Skills. 2009; www.dti.gov.uk/quality/tqm.
14. Pentecost D. Quality management: the human factor. *Euro Particip Mon.* 1991; 8–10.
15. Office of Government Commerce. 2009; www.ogc.gov.uk/documentation_and templates benefits_realisation_plan_.asp.
16. Department of Health. *High Quality Care for All: NHS Next Stage Review final report.* 2008; www.dh.gov.uk/en/Publicationsandstatistics/Publications/PublicationsPolicy AndGuidance/DH_085825.
17. Connecting for Health. 2009; www.connectingforhealth.nhs.uk/systemsandservices/clindash.
18. Balanced Scorecard Institute. 2009; www.balancedscorecard.org/bscresources.

CHAPTER 2

Assessment tool for evaluating AHP management structures

Fiona Jenkins and Robert Jones

INTRODUCTION

Management arrangements for the AHPs often lack consistency and clarity as they do not comfortably 'fit' organisational structures within trusts. In this chapter, we present our Assessment Tool (Table 2.2) for use in evaluating AHP management and organisational structures in the context of quality, effective, efficient and economical service provision. We believe that the proposed Tool is unique in that it can be used to evaluate a wide range of management functions of AHP services.

The Tool has been constructed using evidence-based information from our combined research spanning more than two decades, which has provided a valuable and rich source of data on AHP managers' roles, responsibilities, and duties, together with the views of postholders regarding the management and organisational structures in which they work. Our research has also included comprehensive literature reviews and investigation of organisational models internationally. The Tool has been developed primarily to assess AHP structures in the UK and the terminology used reflects the UK NHS, although it is designed to be transferable to a range of health systems worldwide; it has been reviewed and used by AHP colleagues in the UK Ireland and New Zealand.

The Tool assesses AHP management structures under 10 management *Domains* that were identified from our research. The 10 Domains are:

1 strategic management
2 clinical governance
3 human resource management
4 clinical/professional requirements

5 operational/service management
6 resource management
7 information management
8 education
9 commissioning
10 service improvement/redesign.

The Domains are not listed in any particular priority order.

APPLICATION OF THE *TOOL*

The Tool may be used in two ways. First, the current AHP service is assessed using the scoring sheet. Each management Domain has several sub-domains or Elements that are scored individually using a 'traffic light' scoring mechanism. When all the Elements of the Domain have been traffic light scored, comments and conclusions are recorded. All 10 Domains are assessed in this way.

On completion of the scoring, the results are analysed, enabling AHP managers to determine strengths and weaknesses of the current management and organisational arrangements, how structure impacts on this, and, importantly, how the existing management arrangements facilitate or impede the AHP services in providing high-quality, responsive patient care. This enables managers to determine which Domains of the service:

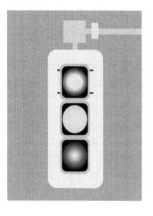

• function as near as possible to optimal
  levels (green traffic lights)
• function less satisfactorily (amber traffic lights)
• function unsatisfactorily (red traffic lights).

If there is an initiative within an organisation to review or change management structures, the AHP manager can use the Tool to score the 10 Domains and individual Elements to assess the likely impact on the service organisation and stakeholders. A comparison between the existing and proposed management structures would then be possible, enabling conclusions to be drawn and constructive dialogue to take place with senior managers and commissioners about the likely advantages and disadvantages of the proposed new arrangements.

SCORING SYSTEM: ASSESSMENT TOOL
FOR AHP MANAGEMENT MODELS

We have designed the Tool to assess strengths and weakness of different management models. It can be used to assess management arrangements already in place and proposals for new arrangements. The two management models (existing system and proposed new system) may then be compared.

The Assessment Tool is constructed in tabular form using a separate box for each Domain (*see* Table 2.1, which illustrates a completed example assessment template for one Domain). Each Domain is numbered: for example, Domain 1—Strategic Management, Domain 2—Clinical Governance, and so on. The Elements within each Domain are also numbered, with space for comments to be recorded if desired. A green, amber, or red score is allocated as appropriate and totalled at the end of each Domain. Following this there are text boxes for comments and conclusions about the Domain.

The Assessment Tool is appropriate for evaluating both individual AHP services—unidisciplinary—and clusters of AHP services where these are managed as one large grouping. There are 10 management Domains, under which the Elements are listed. Not all Elements will apply to all services, and therefore these may be left unmarked. Some Elements apply to more than one Domain, for example, workforce planning, which appears in more than one Domain.

Example

Domain 1 comprises 10 Elements. The traffic light scoring system is completed where:
- Red = No, unable to fulfil this function, unsatisfactory (<25%)
- Amber = Only partially able to fulfil this function
- Green = Yes, able to fulfil this function, satisfactory (>80%).

Comments are made in the element boxes, traffic light scores are totalled, then comments and an overall conclusion about the satisfactoriness or otherwise of the *Domain* are entered in the box at the end of the *Domain*.

We recommend that a separate assessment *pro forma* be used to evaluate each possible or proposed management model.

CONCLUSION

Our overarching objective in developing this Assessment Tool has been to ensure—as far as possible—that AHP management arrangements, structures, and service organisations are focused on infrastructures that facilitate and support provision of the best possible outcomes for our patients, the service providers themselves, and the organisations in which they work.

Change is constant in healthcare and it is essential that we contribute proactively to the process in order to improve services without compromising the legitimate goals of those providing the services, ensuring as best we can that any changes proposed are in the best interests of patient care, are successful, and are good value for the money. There is no simple 'right' or 'one way' of configuring AHP services; however, it is intended that the Assessment Tool will be helpful to those AHP managers and others to evaluate their current services or proposed restructuring and changes.

So often we hear of restructuring that takes place without proper consideration of the likely advantages and disadvantages, or put forward on the basis of 'politics' or 'ownership agendas' of particular organisations or managers. Sometimes, this takes place without proper consideration of how services might be structured to provide optimum high-quality clinical outcomes, appropriate care pathways, patient flows, development for staff, economies of scale, 'critical mass', elimination of duplication, excellent communication and networking, and many others. The Assessment Tool incorporates a 'big picture' overview and it is evidence based, informed by research and detailed studies of the available literature and examination of a wide range of models—some in place, and some theoretical.

There are approximately 214 000 registrants in the 15 professions within the remit of the Health Professions Council in the UK and a large number of support staff in a wide variety of roles. This represents a very significant percentage of healthcare provision and use of resources. This workforce undertakes many millions of healthcare interventions and patient contacts every year. It is essential, therefore, that decisions about management arrangements, structures, and organisation of these services are evaluated using a methodical approach. Our Assessment Tool may be used to contribute to this process.

Table 2.1 Completed example template of the assessment tool

	Red	Amber	Green
1 Strategic management domain			
Mark and comment on each element answering this question: ***Do the management arrangements enable effective:***			
1.1 Contribution to local development process for the whole service *Comments: Yes, fully engaged in making development-planning recommendations for whole service.*			✓
1.2 Medium- and long-term planning and service development for whole service (strategic plan for whole service for one to three years) *Comments: Have a plan for two years ahead, not three years.*		✓	
1.3 Contribution to the regional workforce plan for the professional group(s) *Comments: No, not involved in input to workforce plan for my service, HR do the regional return without my input.*	✓		
1.4 Medium- to long-term workforce planning for the whole service (for one to three years) *Comments: Yes, I have a workforce plan developed within the service.*			✓

Table 2.1 Completed example template of the assessment tool (*Continued*)

	Red	Amber	Green
1.5 Non-fragmented service through effective strategic management of whole service *Comments: Provide both acute and community services, staff managed as one group.*			✓
1.6 Clear lines of accountability for the whole service(s) (both management and professional accountability) *Comments: All staff have one management and professional line of accountability.*			✓
1.7 Management authority for the whole service (s) (full and equitable management authority) *Comments: Limited management authority in community services, locality managers hold staffing and training budgets in several areas, which limits management authority.*		✓	
1.8 Management responsibility for the whole service(s) (full and equitable management responsibility) *Comments: Full management responsibility for acute hospital-based staff, but not for all community staff.*		✓	
1.9 Initiation and management and monitoring of service-level agreements (where these are in place) *Comments: Do not have any SLAs in place but should have as we provide services in other organisations.*	✓		
1.10 Strategic development and partnership working with other organisations such as social services and education *Comments: Yes, have well-established senior-level strategic mechanisms.*			✓
1.11 Initiation and management and monitoring of external contracts (where these are in place) *Comments: Yes, have contracts with care homes that I initiated and monitor.*			✓
1.12 Implementation of government policies and initiatives across the entire service(s) *Comments: Have authority to do this in only part of the service.*		✓	
1.13 Comprehensive strategic overview for the profession(s) to be fully engaged at the strategic level *Comments: Head of service not engaged at strategic level, only input is from band 7 clinicians.*	✓		
Traffic light totals	**3**	**4**	**6**
Overall domain conclusion: Mostly positive, however, room to improve strategic workforce planning, develop SLAs, and engage head of service. Community-based staff have less access to training funds as these are held by the locality managers and less flexibility with staff management as staff budgets are held by community services.			

Table 2.2 Assessment of management structures: the assessment tool

Assessment criteria	Red	Amber	Green
1 Strategic management domain			
Mark and comment on each element answering this question: **Do the management arrangements enable:**			
1.1 Effective contribution to local planning process for the whole service *Comments:*			
1.2 Medium and long-term planning and service development for the whole service (strategic plan for whole service for one to three years) *Comments:*			
1.3 Contribution to the regional workforce plan for the professional group(s) *Comments:*			
1.4 Medium- to long-term workforce planning for the whole service (for one to three years) *Comments:*			
1.5 Non-fragmentation of the service through effective strategic management of the whole service *Comments:*			
1.6 Clear lines of accountability for the whole service(s) (both management and professional accountability) *Comments:*			
1.7 Effective management authority for the whole service(s) (full and equitable management authority) *Comments:*			
1.8 Effective management responsibility for the whole service(s) (full and equitable management responsibility) *Comments:*			
1.9 Initiation and management and monitoring of service-level agreements (where these are in place) *Comments:*			
1.10 Strategic development and partnership working with other organisations such as social services and education *Comments:*			
1.11 Initiation and management and monitoring of external contracts (where these are in place) *Comments:*			
1.12 Implementation of government policies and initiatives across the whole service(s) *Comments:*			

Table 2.2 Assessment of management structures: the assessment tool (*Continued*)

Assessment criteria	Red	Amber	Green
1.13 Strategic overview for the profession(s) to be comprehensive *Comments:*			
Traffic light totals			
Overall domain conclusion:			
2 Clinical governance domain			
Mark and comment on each element answering this question: ***Do the management arrangements enable:***			
2.1 The provision of effective patient-centred services— including cross-boundary working to deliver care pathways and the involvement of service users in planning and service evaluation *Comments:*			
2.2 Effective implementation of evidence-based practice equally across the whole service(s) *Comments:*			
2.3 Consistent management of research and development activity across the whole service(s) *Comments:*			
2.4 Consistent management of clinical audit across the whole service(s) *Comments:*			
2.5 Effective management of service risk across the whole service(s) *Comments:*			
2.6 Effective management of health and safety across the whole service(s) *Comments:*			
2.7 Management of equitable staff education and training across the whole service(s) *Comments:*			
2.8 Management of efficient, equitable staffing and staff management across the whole service(s) *Comments:*			
2.9 Effective communication across the whole service(s) *Comments:*			

(*Continued*)

Table 2.2 Assessment of management structures: the assessment tool (*Continued*)

Assessment criteria	Red	Amber	Green
2.10 Rapid and equitable management of and response to complaints across the whole service(s) *Comments:*			
Traffic light totals			
Overall domain conclusion:			
3 Human resource management			
Mark and comment on each element answering this question: ***Do the management arrangements enable:***			
3.1 Effective staff recruitment to all grades and all specialties throughout the service(s) *Comments:*			
3.2 Career progression opportunities and succession planning across the entire service(s) *Comments:*			
3.3 Flexibility of staff deployment across the service(s) to cover absence, sickness, leave, etc. *Comments:*			
3.4 Flexible working arrangements such as the provision of seven-day working *Comments:*			
3.5 Uniform application of grievance and disciplinary procedures across the entire service(s) *Comments:*			
3.6 Consistent application of HR policies and procedures for all staff across the entire service(s) *Comments:*			
3.7 Equitable and consistent application of the Agenda for Change across the entire service(s) *Comments:*			
3.8 Equitable implementation of Improving Working Lives across the entire service(s) *Comments:*			
3.9 Appropriate high-level professional responsibility and authority to recruit and dismiss staff across the organisation *Comments:*			

Table 2.2 Assessment of management structures: the assessment tool (*Continued*)

Assessment criteria	Red	Amber	Green
3.10 Nationally required regulatory procedures (HPC) to be implemented and monitored across the whole service (s) *Comments:*			
3.11 Workforce planning for whole service(s), including appropriate skill mix and input to workforce commissioning procedures *Comments:*			
Traffic light totals			
Overall domain conclusion:			
4 Clinical professional requirements			
Mark and comment on each element answering this question: ***Do the management arrangements enable:***			
4.1 Appropriate high-level clinical and professional leadership and consultancy across the whole service(s) *Comments:*			
4.2 'Critical mass' of staff—a broad range of grades and specialisms to be in place across the whole service(s) *Comments:*			
4.3 Effective non-fragmented service provision and good communication across organisations *Comments:*			
4.4 Professionally relevant and consistent development and implementation of knowledge and skills framework profiles across service(s) *Comments:*			
4.5 Professionally relevant and consistent personal development plans and CPD in place across entire service(s) *Comments:*			
4.6 A range of appropriate post-registration education to meet staff needs, with expertise in all clinical specialties across service(s) *Comments:*			
4.7 Comprehensive in-service training and education to meet the needs of all staff *Comments:*			

(*Continued*)

Table 2.2 Assessment of management structures: the assessment tool (*Continued*)

Assessment criteria	Red	Amber	Green
4.8 Effective management development and relevant professional mentoring across the entire service(s) *Comments:*			
4.9 The management of career progression and succession planning on an equitable basis throughout the entire service(s) *Comments:*			
4.10 Effective leadership development across the entire service(s) *Comments:*			
4.11 Appropriate professional supervision and support to be in place for all staff across the service(s) *Comments:*			
4.12 Clinical supervision systems in place for staff *Comments:*			
4.13 Appropriate supervision and support for newly qualified staff, including staff rotations across specialties in all core areas across the whole service(s) *Comments:* .			
4.14 Undergraduate (student) clinical placements across all core areas *Comments:*			
4.15 Undergraduate clinical placements across specialist areas *Comments:*			
4.16 Effective implementation of evidence-based practice across the entire service(s) *Comments:*			
4.17 Implementation, consistent use, and monitoring of appropriate validated outcome measures across the entire service(s) *Comments:*			
4.18 Design and implementation of protocols, procedures, and guidelines (managerial and clinical) for the whole service(s) *Comments:*			
4.19 Consistent implementation of national guidelines and policies across the entire service(s) *Comments:*			
4.20 Effective clinical and managerial engagement of appropriate staff in national, regional and local professional for a. *Comments:*			

Table 2.2 Assessment of management structures: the assessment tool (*Continued*)

Assessment criteria	Red	Amber	Green
4.21 High-quality record-keeping systems, in line with legal and professional standards, throughout the entire service(s) *Comments:*			
Traffic light totals			
Overall domain conclusion:			
5 Operational/service management			
Mark and comment on each element answering this question: ***Do the management arrangements enable:***			
5.1 Effective and efficient use of staff resources - use of time, skills and expertise in all areas across service(s) *Comments:*			
5.2 Effective day-to-day management of clinical staff in all areas of service(s) *Comments:*			
5.3 Appropriate staff deployment in all areas across service(s) – to ensure right skills in the right place *Comments:*			
5.4 The elimination of unnecessary duplication of service provision, expertise and resource use *Comments:*			
5.5 Effective day-to-day management of clinical practice in all areas of service(s) *Comments:*			
5.6 Effective performance management and monitoring of clinical standards of staff across whole service(s) *Comments:*			
5.7 Effective day-to-day management of clinical pathways and vertical integration across all areas of service(s) *Comments:*			
5.8 Continuity for service users between acute hospital and primary care services *Comments:*			
5.9 Effective networking across services/organisations to facilitate non-fragmented patient care *Comments:*			

(*Continued*)

Table 2.2 Assessment of management structures: the assessment tool (*Continued*)

Assessment criteria	Red	Amber	Green
5.10 Effective collaborative working between the service and other agencies such as social, education, voluntary or independent sector *Comments:*			
5.11 Ensure positive interdisciplinary working across organisation(s) *Comments:*			
Traffic light totals			
Overall domain conclusion:			
6 Management of resources			
Mark and comment on each element answering this question: ***Do the management arrangements enable:***			
6.1 High-level professional input, accountability, responsibility, and authority for budget management across the entire service(s) *Comments:*			
6.2 High-level professional input to the budget-setting process for the entire service(s) *Comments:*			
6.3 Active participation in financial planning and monitoring processes throughout the year for the whole service(s) *Comments:*			
6.4 Achievement of economies of scale—economic use of resources (human and financial) throughout the entire service(s) *Comments:*			
6.5 Optimum use of facilities and equipment across the entire service(s) *Comments:*			
6.6 Income-generation projects, including innovative use of NHS facilities across the entire service(s) *Comments:*			
6.7 The most senior AHP manager input to costing and pricing process to ensure consistent application across the entire service(s) *Comments:*			

Table 2.2 Assessment of management structures: the assessment tool (*Continued*)

Assessment criteria	Red	Amber	Green
6.8 Equitable management of AHP charitable trust funds across the entire service(s) where these exist *Comments:*			
6.9 Involvement in capital project planning and management relevant to the entire service(s) *Comments:*			
6.10 Effective mechanisms for procurement and stock control for the entire service(s) *Comments:*			
6.11 Effective input to relevant tendering procedures to be in place *Comments:*			
Traffic light totals			
Overall domain conclusion:			
7 Information management			
Mark and comment on each element answering this question: ***Do the management arrangements enable:***			
7.1 Effective management of clinical and managerial information throughout the service(s) *Comments:*			
7.2 Uniformity of IM&T across the service(s) *Comments:*			
7.3 Proactive input in the development of uniform IM&T across the service(s) *Comments:*			
7.4 Consistent interpretation of information across the entire service(s). *Comments:*			
7.5 Management of timely, accurate, and relevant information across the entire service(s) *Comments:*			
7.6 Consistent data analysis of activity and referral patterns across the entire service(s) *Comments:*			

(*Continued*)

Table 2.2 Assessment of management structures: the assessment tool (*Continued*)

Assessment criteria	Red	Amber	Green
7.7 The application of uniform data sets and coding across the entire service(s) *Comments:*			
7.8 The provision of uniform quality information for patients across the entire service(s) *Comments:*			
7.9 Uniform record-keeping across the service(s) *Comments:*			
7.10 Uniform availability of timely and accurate staffing establishment information for the entire service(s) *Comments:*			
7.11 Uniform availability of timely and accurate budget information for the entire service(s) *Comments:*			
7.12 Uniform collection and analysis of data on activity and throughput across the entire service(s) *Comments:*			
Traffic light totals			
Overall domain conclusion:			
8 Education and training			
Mark and comment on each element answering this question: ***Do the management arrangements enable:***			
8.1 High-level professional input to the region in pre-registration education contract setting and monitoring for the whole service(s) *Comments:*			
8.2 High-level professional input to post-registration education demand forecasting for the entire service(s) *Comments:*			
8.3 High-level professional input to pre-registration education demand forecasting based on service needs for the entire service(s) *Comments:*			
8.4 Budget management for whole service postgraduate education and training to ensure equity and appropriate use of funding across the service(s) *Comments:*			

Table 2.2 Assessment of management structures: the assessment tool (*Continued*)

Assessment criteria	Red	Amber	Green
8.5 The initiation and management of R&D projects across the entire service(s) *Comments:*			
8.6 Implementation of appropriate education and training programmes for support staff across the entire service(s) *Comments:*			
8.7 Higher education institutions to have a clearly identified point of contact for the management of undergraduate placements for the entire service(s) *Comments:*			
8.8 Higher education institutions to have a clearly identified professional senior manager point of contact for input to course evaluation and development *Comments:*			
Traffic light totals			
Overall domain conclusion:			
9 Commissioning/service planning			
Mark and comment on each element answering this question: ***Do the management arrangements enable:***			
9.1 Effective professional senior manager input to the commissioning/planning process for the entire service(s) *Comments:*			
9.2 Effective involvement of service users in evaluation and development of service(s) *Comments:*			
9.3 Management of consistent service-level agreements across the entire service(s) *Comments:*			
9.4 Management of professionally relevant service specifications across the entire service(s) *Comments:*			
9.5 Management of professionally relevant service contracts with non-NHS purchasers, e.g. hospices or voluntary organisations *Comments:*			

(*Continued*)

Table 2.2 Assessment of management structures: the assessment tool (*Continued*)

Assessment criteria	Red	Amber	Green
9.6 Active senior professional management engagement in 'choice' agenda for the entire service(s)(where applicable) *Comments:*			
Traffic light totals			
Overall domain conclusion:			
10 Service improvement and redesign			
Mark and comment on each element answering this question: ***Do the management arrangements enable:***			
10.1 Management, leadership, and implementation of innovative service improvements and redesign across the entire service(s) *Comments:*			
10.2 Development of consultant AHP posts *Comments:*			
10.3 Development of extended scope AHP posts *Comments:*			
10.4 Development of clinical specialist and advanced practitioner AHP posts *Comments:*			
10.5 Introduction of new ways of working across the entire service(s), e.g. seven days a week working *Comments:*			
10.6 Active engagement in multidisciplinary service developments, e.g. stroke service redesign for the entire health community *Comments:*			
10.7 Skill mix review and service re-profiling across the entire service(s) as appropriate *Comments:*			
10.8 Appropriate professional senior management input to the development of new types of posts and generic roles *Comments:*			
10.9 Inclusion of staff of all grades to input to service improvement and innovation *Comments:*			

Table 2.2 Assessment of management structures: the assessment tool (*Continued*)

Assessment criteria	Red	Amber	Green
10.10 Patient/service user engagement in service improvement *Comments:*			
10.11 The introduction of expert patient programmes as appropriate throughout the entire service(s) *Comments:*			
10.12 Involvement of voluntary and public sector organisations in service improvement initiatives across the entire service(s) *Comments:*			
Traffic light totals			
Overall domain conclusion:			

CHAPTER 3

Benchmarking AHP services

Fiona Jenkins and Robert Jones

BENCHMARKING YOUR SERVICE

Benchmarking is an invaluable means of enhancing understanding of your service's performance achieved through making comparisons with other organisations. It demonstrates how your service is performing in relation to similar AHP services and will also indicate whether the full potential of the workforce and other resources is being fully realised. If, as AHP managers, we have no idea what the standards for a wide range of parameters are, we cannot compare to establish the relationship between our organisation and others. Benchmarking is often used as part of service review and for quality improvement initiatives. The technique is a widely used management tool that had its origins in manufacturing industry and is now used in public services, including healthcare.

INTRODUCING OUR AHP BENCHMARKING TOOL

We have developed this AHP benchmarking tool, which can be used by managers to help set standards and monitor whether or not these are being met in terms of workforce, resources, activity, availability, access, and so on. To date, there has been no universally accepted 'validated tool' or process available to AHP managers and their teams to use and undertake this work. In view of this and as a result of our own experience in undertaking service reviews evaluation and consultancy, we recognised that a basic benchmarking process, which is evidence-based, would be helpful to AHP managers and wider healthcare organisations.

Initially the tool included a wide range of specialties, but following piloting and advice received from heads of AHP services and clinicians, we decreased the number of categories included to facilitate ease of completion and opportunity for comparisons to be made. Our benchmarking tool is designed to be objective and a straightforward process, which can either be used to review your own service in isolation, or to make comparisons with aspects of other services, or other services in their entirety. We hope the tool will support and be helpful to AHP managers undertaking benchmarking exercises.

HOW TO USE THE TOOL

Firstly, we set out below data collection forms. This is followed by a set of briefing notes that explain how the process should be completed.

THE BENCHMARKING 'TOOLKIT'

The tool has five sections.
1   Your organisation.
2   Your professional group.
3   Inpatient services.
4   Outpatient services.
5   Community services.

BRIEFING NOTES

The purpose of these briefing notes is to ensure—as far as possible—a consistent and accurate methodology for collecting the data between the provider services participating in benchmarking exercises. Organisations taking part may be widely dispersed across the region, country, or between countries, and there are differing practices and definitions in use in different places. Therefore, uniformity of approach will help to ensure that the data collected enables valid comparisons and consistent interpretation.

It is possible to select only a few categories for benchmarking, or to include the whole service. The more generic categories that are chosen to describe the service, the more likely it will be to find a comparator to benchmark with. Therefore, consider very carefully the categories you select to benchmark. We recognise, for example, that some areas have elderly care wards and in other areas, elderly care is part of general medicine—we have amalgamated this and have one category, general medicine.

We also recognise that different professions have different sub-specialisms, for example, gastroenterology is likely to be a high input for dietitians, but physiotherapists may include this inpatient activity as part of general medicine.

Confidentiality is guaranteed; if your service/organisation wishes to remain anonymous, please indicate on the form. The data collection spreadsheet is divided into five sections.

Table 3.1 Spreadsheet 1: your organisation

Date:

Provider name:

Professional groups being benchmarked:

1.	WTE HPC Reg Staff........	WTE Non-Reg Clinical Staff........	WTE A&C........ Grand total WTE all staff........
2.	WTE HPC Reg Staff........	WTE Non-Reg Clinical Staff........	WTE A&C........ Grand total WTE all staff........
3.	WTE HPC Reg Staff........	WTE Non-Reg Clinical Staff........	WTE A&C........ Grand total WTE all staff........
4.	WTE HPC Reg Staff........	WTE Non-Reg Clinical Staff........	WTE A&C........ Grand total WTE all staff........
5.	WTE HPC Reg Staff........	WTE Non-Reg Clinical Staff........	WTE A&C........ Grand total WTE all staff........
6.	WTE HPC Reg Staff........	WTE Non-Reg Clinical Staff........	WTE A&C........ Grand total WTE all staff........

Contact details for the person completing the form (optional):

Name:

Position:

E-mail address:

Provider type (please tick)**:**

1. Acute Trust

2. Foundation Trust

3. Care Trust

4. Mental Health Trust

5. Combined Acute and Community

6. Tertiary

7. Health Board

8. Other please specify

Catchment population:

Total number of beds in organisation:

Budget for services being benchmarked (list professional groups):

1.	Total Budget = £	Pay Budget = £	Non-Pay Budget = £
2.	Total Budget = £	Pay Budget = £	Non-Pay Budget = £
3.	Total Budget = £	Pay Budget = £	Non-Pay Budget = £
4.	Total Budget = £	Pay Budget = £	Non-Pay Budget = £
5.	Total Budget = £	Pay Budget = £	Non-Pay Budget = £
6.	Total Budget = £	Pay Budget = £	Non-Pay Budget = £

Grand totals: £ £ £

Do you want to keep your organisation's name anonymous? (Yes/No please specify)

SECTION 1 YOUR ORGANISATION—GENERAL INFORMATION

Only one Section 1 form needs filling in per organisation.
- Date: the date the form is completed.
- Provider name: the name of your organisation.
- Professional groups being benchmarked: please list the professions for benchmarking and then insert the WTE HPC reg. staff ... WTE non-reg. clinical staff ... WTE A&C ... grand total WTE all staff ....
- Contact details for the person completing the form: generally the most senior AHP manager in the service. Please give name and e-mail contact, but this may be withheld if you wish.
- Provider type: e.g. Acute Trust, Community Services, Care Trust, Foundation Trust, Tertiary Provider, Integrated Health Board, etc.
- Catchment population for your organisation: please state the population in thousands.
- Total number of beds in the organisation: list the current declared bed stock.
- Budget for services being benchmarked: first list the services being benchmarked, then include the total budget, pay budget, and non-pay budget for all of the professional groups combined and finally add up the columns to give the grand totals.
- Indicate whether you want your organisation's name to be kept anonymous: highlight Yes or No.

NB. Each individual profession will need to complete sections 2–5 inclusive as appropriate.

SECTION 2 YOUR PROFESSIONAL GROUP AND STAFFING
- Total WTE managerial staff: please fill in the boxes that are not shaded as appropriate. For staff with mixed managerial and clinical roles, please include here the approximate WTE of their time assigned to management duties.
- Total WTE clinical staff for your professional group (excluding consultants): this includes every member of staff you employ, working within your organisation.
- Total WTE AHP consultants.
- Total WTE assistant and support staff.
- Total WTE administration and clerical staff.
- Staff from your professional group you provide to other organisations: this would include the staff that you employ and that you may have service-level agreements to provide to another organisation, e.g., rotational staff, hospices, etc.
- Total staff: please add up the rows to give your total staff by band for the staff group.

Table 3.2 Spreadsheet 2: your professional group

Your professional group

	WTE Registered Staff									WTE Non-Registered Staff						Total WTE staff in this group
	Band 5	Band 6	Band 7	Band 8a	Band 8b	Band 8c	Band 8d	Band 9	Director	Band 2	Band 3	Band 4	Band 5	Band 6	Band 7	
Total WTE Managerial Staff HPC Registered																
Total WTE Clinical HPC Registered Staff for your professional group, excluding consultants																
Total WTE AHP consultants																
Total WTE—assistants and support staff																
Total WTE Admin & clerical staff																
Staff from your professional group you provide to other organizations																

Table 3.3 Spreadsheet 3: inpatient services

Your professional group:

Clinical specialities. Select specialties relevant to your profession—see briefing notes.	Beds per specialty	WTE Registered Staff								WTE Non-Registered Staff				Total all staff for specialty	Activity		7 day service Yes/No	Validated clinical outcome measures used? Yes*/No
		Band 5	Band 6	Band 7	Band 8a	Band 8b	Band 8c	Band 8d	Band 9	Band 2	Band 3	Band 4	Band 5		New patients last year	Total contacts last year		
ENT (SALT only)																		
Gastroenterology (Dietetics only)																		
General Medicine (including elderly care)																		
General Surgery																		
HDU																		
Head and neck (Dietetics and SALT only)																		
ITU																		
Emergency admissions																		
Mental health																		
Neurology																		
Obstetrics and Gynaecology																		
Oncology																		
Paediatrics																		
Palliative care																		
SCBU																		
Stroke unit																		
Trauma and Orthopaedic																		
Other 1. Please specify																		
Other 2. Please specify																		
Other 3. Please specify																		
Other 4. Please specify																		
Other 5. Please specify																		

*Please list validated outcome measures used.

SECTION 3 INPATIENT SERVICES

An inpatient service is defined as:

One where patients (clients) occupy beds overnight as part of their episode of care. This may be in acute or community settings and in health or social care.

The list of specialities is not exhaustive, but it is hoped that most therapy services will be able to group their total inpatient activity under several of the categories listed. It is not intended for every speciality to be used by every professional group.

Where highly specialist or tertiary services are provided, please list them in the 'other' category—though this may make it more difficult to benchmark.

- Your professional group: name the professional group you are reporting information for.
- Beds per specialty: for the specialties you are proving data for, please indicate the current number of beds in the unshaded boxes.
- WTE registered staff: i.e., staff registered with the HPC.
- WTE non-registered staff: i.e., assistants and clinical support staff do not include clerical staff in this section.
- Total staff: please add up the rows to give your total staff for the specialty.
- New patients last year: total number of new patients for the last financial year.
- Total contacts last year: total face-to-face contacts for the last financial year.
- Seven-day service yes/no: this includes routine working, even if only for part of the day and not an 'on-call' service.
- Validated clinical outcome measures used: please identify at the bottom of the sheet the names of the validated outcome measures used.
- Clinical specialties: for each of these broadly defined clinical specialties, enter the relevant data in each column. Some clinical specialties listed will not require detailed benchmark scrutiny for every professional group, e.g., gastroenterology is likely to be pertinent to dietetic services, whereas physiotherapy may group this service as part of general medical services. Similarly, it is unlikely that podiatry services will input to ITU regularly. It is anticipated that data will be provided for a wide range of specialties for each profession.
- Other please specify: if your inpatient service is very different from one in the list, e.g., tertiary service, cardiothoracic, or neurosurgery, please identify it and provide data.
- Day surgery: provide data for therapy input to day surgery services, i.e., where there is no overnight stay.
- Total staff: please add up columns to give your total staff by band.

SECTION 4 OUTPATIENT SERVICES

An outpatient is someone who attends a hospital or clinic for treatment that does not require an overnight stay.

Table 3.4 Spreadsheet 4: outpatient services

Your professional group:

Specialities. Select specialties relevant to your profession—see briefing notes.	WTE Registered Staff								WTE Non-Registered Staff				Total all staff for specialty	Is group treatment included in this specialty? Yes/No	Activity				Validated clinical outcome measures used? Yes*/No
	Band 5	Band 6	Band 7	Band 8a	Band 8b	Band 8c	Band 8d	Band 9	Band 2	Band 3	Band 4	Band 5			Average no. new patients/week per WTE	New patients last year	Total contacts last year	DNA %	
A&E																			
Cardiac rehab																			
Communication SALT only																			
Diabetes (Dietetics and Podiatry only)																			
Dysfluency (SALT only)																			
Fracture clinic																			
Gait clinics																			
Gastroenterology (Dietetics only)																			
Hand therapy																			
Head and neck (Dietetics and SALT only)																			
Hydrotherapy (physio only)																			
Musculoskeletal																			
Neurology (excluding stroke)																			
Nutritional support (Dietetics only)																			
Occupational Health																			
Orthotics																			
Paediatrics																			
Pain management																			
Palliative care																			
Pulmonary Rehab																			
Rheumatology																			
Stroke																			
Voice (SALT only)																			
Wheelchairs and seating																			
Women s/Men's health																			
Other 1. Please specify																			
Other 2. Please specify																			
Other 3. Please specify																			

*Please list validated outcome measures used.

This section is to gather information on patients who meet this definition. This could include both adult and children's services, and may be in primary or secondary care and normally in a healthcare setting.

The list of specialities is not exhaustive, and is intended to give a reasonable level of specialisation for each profession, but also recognises that to list every therapy sub-speciality would be an exhaustive process. It is not intended for every speciality to be used by every professional group.

Where highly specialist or tertiary services are provided, please list them in the 'other' category—this may make it more difficult to benchmark, so only use when really necessary.

- Your professional group: name the professional group you are reporting information for.
- WTE registered staff: i.e., staff registered with the HPC.
- WTE non-registered staff: i.e., assistants and clinical support staff, do not include clerical staff in this section.
- Total staff: please add up rows to give your total staff for the specialty.
- Group treatment: answer yes or no for each specialty.
- Average number new patients/week per WTE: where staff are set a target number of new patients per week, please enter this number for each speciality that this applies to.
- New patients last year: total number of new patients for the last financial year.
- Total contacts last year: total face-to-face contacts for the last financial year.
- DNA per cent: this includes all DNA and UTA for first and follow-up appointments as a percentage of all appointments.
- Validated clinical outcome measures used: please identify at the bottom of the sheet the names of the validated outcome measures used.
- Outpatient specialties: for each of these broadly defined specialties, enter the relevant data in each column. Some specialties listed will not be relevant to all professional groups, e.g., dysfluency is likely to be only a speech and language therapy specialty, whereas wheelchair and seating clinics may be pertinent for both physiotherapy and occupational therapy. It is anticipated that data will be provided for a wide range of specialties for each profession, but not each and every one.
- Other please specify: if your outpatient service is different from one in the list, please identify it and provide data, this may make it more difficult to benchmark, so only use when really necessary.

SECTION 5 COMMUNITY SERVICES

Community services are those therapy services that are provided away from hospital premises and are neither inpatient services nor outpatient. Examples would

Table 3.5 Spreadsheet 5: community services

Your professional group:

Specialities. Select specialties relevant to your profession—see briefing notes.	WTE Registered Staff								WTE Non-Registered Staff				Total all staff for specialty	Is group treatment included in this specialty? Yes/No	Activity				Validated clinical outcome measures used? Yes*/No
	Band 5	Band 6	Band 7	Band 8a	Band 8b	Band 8c	Band 8d	Band 9	Band 2	Band 3	Band 4	Band 5			New patients last year	Total contacts last year	7 day service Yes/No	DNA%	
Community hospital rehabilitation ward																			
Domiciliary adult																			
Domiciliary paediatric																			
Intermediate Care																			
Learning Disabilities																			
Mental Health																			
Neuro rehab (excluding stroke)																			
Paediatric																			
Social Services																			
Stroke																			
Other 1. Please specify																			
Other 2. Please specify																			
Other 3. Please specify																			
Other 4. Please specify																			
Other 5. Please specify																			

*Please list validated outcome measures used.

include services provided to education and a range of community-based facilities such as GP surgeries, community clinics, and children's centres.

- Your professional group: name the professional group you are reporting information for.
- WTE registered staff: i.e., staff registered with the HPC.
- WTE non-registered staff: i.e., assistants and clinical support staff, do not include clerical staff in this section.
- Total staff: please add up rows to give your total staff for the specialty.
- Group treatment: answer yes or no for each specialty.
- New patients last year: total number of new patients for the last financial year.
- Total contacts last year: total face-to-face contacts for the last financial year.
- Seven-day service yes/no: this includes routine working, even if only for part of the day and not an 'on-call' service.
- DNA per cent: this includes all DNA and UTA for first and follow-up appointments as a percentage of all appointments.
- Validated clinical outcome measures used: please identify at the bottom of the sheet the names of the validated outcome measures used.
- Community types: for each of these broadly defined types, enter the relevant data in each column. Some listed will not be relevant to all professional groups. It is anticipated that data will be provided for a wide range of specialties for each profession, but not necessarily every one.
- Other please specify: if your community service is different from one in the list, please identify it and provide data; this may make it more difficult to benchmark, so only use when really necessary.

REFERENCE

1. www.jjconsulting.org.uk.

CHAPTER 4

Time is money—how do we spend it? Analysing staff activity

Robert Jones and Fiona Jenkins

INTRODUCTION

AHP managers need to have an accurate picture of workforce activity: the through-put, exactly what work is undertaken, who does it, where it happens, and what sort of service or interventions are provided. A thorough understanding of work activity is essential to service and workforce planning, development of staffing profiles for specific programmes such as the consultant-led 18 weeks pathway and service redesign, and for a wide range of other purposes, such as for costing and pricing, evidence-based staff deployment, contract development, service-level agreements, capacity and demand management, and payment by results. Staff activity analysis also facilitates evidence-based service development and strategy, enabling critical evaluation of different staff activities to support specific projects. This technique is essential for understanding management and administrative inputs and supporting analysis of patterns of work for capacity and demand management. If carried out in collaboration with colleagues from other organisations, the approach can also be used for benchmarking exercises. Activity analysis is also important in monitoring and supporting a range of clinical governance parameters.

Activity analysis is a method of sampling volumes and types of activity undertaken by AHP staff in all grades and specialties on a regular 'snapshot' basis, using a sample activity data collection process based on a template form used for data extract to be input to a programme for reporting and subsequent analysis and interpretation. The different components of patient-related work and non-patient care need to be understood for effective and efficient service provision and management in the increasingly business environment.

This approach has been used in our services and the data obtained used for management and clinical purposes and for benchmarking between locations.

TIPS FOR IMPLEMENTATION
- Ensure the data collection form is fully tested and piloted.
- Involve all team members.
- Computer support and analysis is essential.
- Forward planning for the sample enquiry is important.
- Thorough teaching of definitions of the data items.
- It is essential to share results and outcomes with all teams taking part in the sample.

Box 4.1 Therapy services activity sample form: briefing notes.
Understanding staff activity and the way we spend our working hours is important for management, clinical, and financial purposes and when developing new services and redesigning current ones. The activity sample can be run as a 'snapshot', for example, a week or for a more comprehensive analysis, a 13-week quarter can be used, doing one day per week, that is, week 1 Monday, week 2 Tuesday, and so on. A consistent approach to completing the form is needed, so these briefing notes should be shared with all staff who are to undertake the survey. The form is divided into four main sections:
1   general information
2   patient-related activity
3   non-patient-related activity
4   about your contracted working hours and caseloads
   - each member of staff completes a new form on each day of the activity sample whether working that day or not
   - the main activity sample takes place Monday to Friday inclusive, but members of staff working at the weekend will also be requested to complete forms for those days
   - the form should be completed by HPC-registered staff and assistants.

Part 1—general information
Professional group: the AHP professional group of which you are a member (including assistants), e.g. occupational therapy, dietetics, or physiotherapy.

Date: the date on which the form is completed. All forms must be completed on the same day as the activity takes place. It is best to do this as you go through the day to be sure of accuracy.

Site: this is where you are working, e.g. DGH, community hospital, domiciliary, or special school. If you work in more than one site on one day, a new form should be completed for each site.

Location: the place within your organisation where the interventions take place; e.g. wards, physiotherapy department, podiatry clinics, and patients' homes.

Clinician code: the individual staff code (whatever is used within the organisation for your personal identifier.

Band: agenda for change grade.

Your post name/rotation: e.g. clinical specialist in … Band 5 inpatient rotation, outpatient department assistant.

Absent? Reason: why you are not working today, e.g. annual leave, part-time do not work today, study leave, and/or sick.

Part 2—patient-related activity

Please enter hours and minutes spent on each activity accurately:
- face-to-face contact with individual patients
- face-to-face contact with patients in groups
- telephone contacts with patients, relatives, and carers
- ward rounds
- case conferences
- liaison with other services related to patient care
- administrative work related to patient care, e.g. record-keeping
- home assessment visits with or without the patient in attendance
- clinics
- other patient-related activity to capture others not included above (must be strictly patient-related).

Part 3—non-patient-related activity

Please enter hours and minutes spent on each activity accurately:
- liaison with other services, not related to patient care, could be for a wide range of reasons
- administration; not patient-related, e.g. sending out appointments
- management duties; all work involved in service management or management duties within the organisation
- study leave—you are on study leave yourself
- travel; in the community, between sites or locations, walking the corridors
- staff and team meetings
- in-service education/training; attendance (not leading or presenting)
- teaching and training; when you are leading, presenting or giving this for
- your own professional group
- students

- others
- clinical supervision; providing or attending
- other non-patient-related activities not captured above.

Part 4—about your contracted hours and caseload

- *Your contracted working hours today:* the number of hours you are contracted to work that day, if part time and not working that day, indicate this.
- *Number of group sessions you have done today.*
- *Number of patients on your caseload today:* how many patients did you see or should you have seen, including did not attends or unable to attends (DNA or UTA).
- The total number of patients you have on your overall caseload; how many patients are registered to be seen by you at present.

THERAPY SERVICES ACTIVITY SAMPLE *PRO FORMA*

Professional group: _____

Date	Site	Location	Clinician code	Band	Your post name/ rotation	Absent? Reason

Activity level	Hours	Minutes
Patient-related		
Face-to-face contact (individual)		
Face-to-face contacts (group)		
Telephone contacts with patient or relative		
Ward rounds		
Case conferences		
Liaison with other services—related to patient care		
Administration—patient-related		
Home assessment visits		
Clinics		
Other (patient-related)		

Non-patient-related				
Liaison with other services—not related to patient				
Administration—not patient-related				
Management duties				
Study leave				
Travel				
Staff/team meetings				
In-service training/education				
Teaching/training		Your professional group		
"	"	Students		
"	"	Other		
Clinical supervision				
Other (non-patient-related)				
Your contracted working hours today				
Number of group sessions you have done today				
Number of patients on your caseload today				
The total number of patients currently on your caseload				

EXAMPLE OF REPORTS FROM ACTIVITY SAMPLE

The activity sample data can be analysed and the results shown in tabular or graphical formats as shown in Figures 4.1 to 4.3.

This is the aggregated activity for both patient-related and non-patient-related activity. These can be broken down to look at any specific parameter and make comparisons with any of the others. This type of analysis is an important and powerful tool and needs to be used in association with qualitative measures. By understanding the way that staff read spend their time and the division between patient contact time and non-patient contact time, the manager is able to workforce plan effectively to ensure efficient staffing.

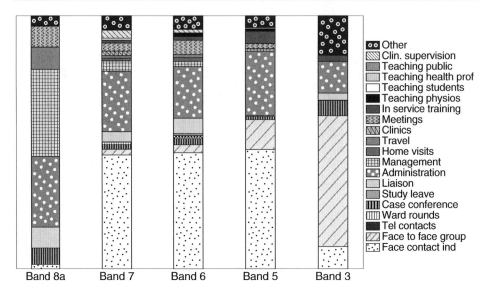

Figure 4.1 Sub-division of staff time by staff band

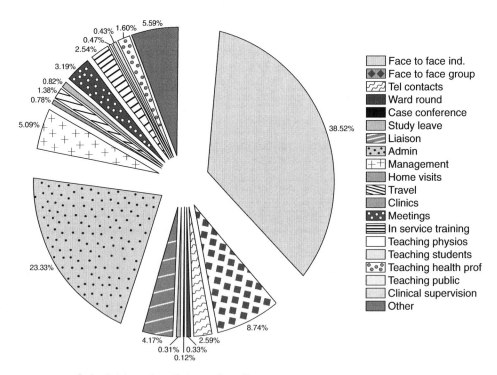

Figure 4.2 Sub-division of staff time; all staff

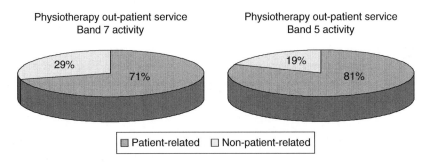

Physiotherapy out-patient service
Band 7 activity

Physiotherapy out-patient service
Band 5 activity

Patient-related   Non-patient-related

Figure 4.3 Comparison of outpatient staff: patient-related to non-patient-related activity by Band 5 and Band 7, physiotherapy outpatient service

Summary

Information management is an essential aspect of AHP management. IM&T offers many benefits to AHP managers, clinicians, and service users, including the following:

- support to strategic and operational management
- support to good business and staff management
- identification of trends
- warning of potential adverse events
- more effective and efficient record-keeping
- better management of patient care
- development of and access to the evidence base
- audit, research, and development.

Whether the service is in primary or secondary care, the private or other sectors, management of the service directly impacts on the quality of care provided. Information management and technology are essential tools to support all elements of quality management to enable service effectiveness and efficiency, management of change, and service redesign. The effective use of data to manage services enables managers to contribute fully to business processes, performance management, and clinical governance.

Information is power, and in the 21st century, all AHP managers and leaders must be increasingly involved in the use of IM&T for current purposes and future development. In order to thrive—or even survive—it is imperative that we have robust information management systems.

CHAPTER 5

Principles for computerised information systems for AHP services

Robert Jones and Fiona Jenkins

INTRODUCTION

AHP managers facing the clinical requirements and the demands of preparing service specifications, business plans, service-level agreements (SLAs), tendering documentation, pricing and costing mechanisms, capacity management including supply and demand, activity, outcomes, caseloads, case mix, and skill mix must be proactive in the development and/or choice of relevant information systems and wider information community.

Not only is this important in its own right, but it is crucial in the wider context of AHP managerial responsibility and clinical autonomy that could be undermined if these services were treated as an 'add-on' to other services such as nursing. The AHP input to patient care is wide-ranging and complex and differs from other services and, therefore, AHP managers must be involved in contributing their specific expertise, managerial and clinical requirements, and management and business needs.

In order to be able to achieve all this—to be able to show what we are doing and how much of it, how effective and efficient it is, and what it all costs—AHPs need powerful computerised information systems capable of bringing together managerial and clinical information.

IM&T is crucial in an ever-increasing business-minded NHS in which the clinical requirements for data and information systems support are paramount. When considering which computerised systems might be suitable for AHP services or contributing to development and specification the principles that we set out below form a useful checklist.

PRINCIPLES FOR COMPUTERISED INFORMATION SYSTEMS FOR AHP SERVICES

1 **Information use.**

   All information collected should be for identified and agreed use. Computerised information systems should provide information required for:
   - clinical, managerial and business purposes within AHP services locally, regionally, and nationally
   - the employing organisation
   - commissioners/planners and all other service purchasers.

2 **Local 'ownership'.**

   The computerised information system should be specific to the clinical and managerial needs of AHP services locally:
   - systems should be 'owned' by the AHP services using them locally, and part of the wider computer system within the organisation
   - information contained within the system is 'owned' by the AHP services and the organisation
   - AHPs should be involved in the choice of appropriate information systems for their service.

3 **Computer hardware.**

   AHP services should have appropriate hardware to support their information systems, and the hardware must:
   - have the capacity to handle the quantity of data required at present and be capable of expansion to meet future needs
   - be capable of supporting a wide variety of applications
   - be capable of supporting a variety of input devices and terminals, including adaptive equipment for sensory-impaired users
   - be compatible with hardware used by other services and departments locally
   - be capable of supporting a variety of data collection modes such as data collection in 'real' time, bar coding, personal digital assistants (PDAs), paper systems, retrospective input, and so on
   - operate at the highest speed commensurate with the size of the information system locally
   - be capable of processing data in 'real' time and batch modes.

4 **Computer software.**

   Computer software for AHP information systems should be appropriate to clinical and managerial practice, and the software must:
   - be specific to AHP managerial and clinical requirements
   - be compatible with other programmes used locally in order to facilitate interfacing
   - enable archiving and retrieval of archived data

- interface easily with other programmes such as Microsoft packages, programmes for clinical purposes, and other databases
- interface with specialist software for sensory-impaired users
    - be capable of updating in line with changing requirements
    - be designed to accommodate SNOMED, ICD, and other coding systems.

5 **System security.**

AHP systems must be secure so as to protect the confidentiality of patients, staff, and others about whom data are held:
- data must be collected, processed, and stored within the requirements of data protection legislation
- entry to the AHP system must be governed by a system of passwords
- staff must log off from computer equipment when not using it
- there must be full backup of data on a daily basis.

6 **Data collection.**

All data collected by AHPs should—whenever possible—be a by-product of clinical practice:
- all patient intervention data items are collected once only if possible
- all data collected by AHPs should be for identified and agreed use
- the data system must facilitate the collection, processing, and reporting of locally agreed clinical and managerial information as well as that required regionally and nationally—it must be possible to report on all parameters input to the system
- the system should facilitate the collection, processing, and reporting of information about the use of AHP resources inpatient activity and non-patient-related activity
- data input to systems may be undertaken by clerical, clinical, or managerial staff.

7 **Reporting.**

The computer system must be capable of producing standard and ad hoc reports for AHP clinical, managerial, research, and business purposes, as well as meeting the agreed requirements of others:
- the system must be able to produce reports to support a wide range of business processes, such as service-line reporting, costing and pricing, referral to treatment time (RTT) reporting, external contract requirements, staff activity, and throughput, capacity, and demand
- the system must be able to produce reports to support a wide range of clinical processes, such as audit, research requirements, clinical case loads, case mix, and outcome measurement
- computer reports must be available to AHP managers and clinicians as and when required

- reports are easily accessible from the system in a variety of modes; tabular, bar charts, pie charts, spreadsheets, and so on
- the system should facilitate the design and generation of ad hoc reports as well as standard reports by AHP managers and clinicians as well as others within the organisation.

8 **Service agreements.**
There must be service agreements with computer companies supplying the AHP system:

- there must be service agreements for the computer software with agreed 'call-out' and support response times
- agreements should include, for example, systems failure, maintenance, support, troubleshooting, and further developments
- it is helpful if there is a user group attended by the software company that the AHP manager can participate in.

9 **Computer system documentation.**
There must be full documentation for the software:

- comprehensive manual on the computerised information system software use
- user manuals
- coding manuals
- report templates.

10 **Staff training.**
Training at all levels on use of the system must be provided:

- training must be provided for clerical and reception staff
- training must be provided for AHP staff.

CHAPTER 6

Functions for Allied Health Professions' record systems

Margaret Hastings

INFORMATION MANAGEMENT

IT supports the real requirements of clinical records, which is information capture and sharing. Identifying the information needs before specifying a system will make it easier for IT to find a solution that meets clinical recording needs.

Table 6.1 Functions for record systems to support AHP clinical recording

Function	Does the system … ?
Patient identification	Auto-populate with demographic information?
	Use unique patient identifier (UPI) based numbering?
	Search on a variety of fields?
	Have links to required external agencies, e.g. NHS care record, birth, death registration?
	Provide linkage between patients, e.g. families?
User identification	Provide secure authentication and access controls?
	Provide positive staff identification linked to registration bodies?
	Allow user demographics with user configurability?
	Have security services including encryption?
Clinical information capture	Allow multi-device support?
	Allow multi-modality support—text, voice, image, and annotation?
	Accommodate digital input devices?
	Allow telemetry?
	Allow 'sticky notes'/Post-its?
	Allow wireless access?
	Allow mobile device download and synchronisation?

(Continued)

Table 6.1 Functions for record systems to support AHP clinical recording (*Continued*)

Function	Does the system ... ?
Care planning and pathways	Allow multidisciplinary views of care plans?
	Provide timelines to oversee care?
	Allow pathways to be developed to follow best practice?
	Provide structured records and clinical templates for care planning?
Workflow management and scheduling	Provide full clinic management requirements?
	Provide complex booking?
	Provide appointment management and outcome?
	Record procedures and interventions to meet regulatory body requirements?
	Schedule user-specific to-do lists and reminders?
Communication	Provide secure clinical messaging/access to messaging systems?
	Provide alerts to other service providers delivering care?
	Provide external, multi-modality telecommunications support for remote consultation/telemedicine?
Screening	Provide call-recall, surveillance for patients on screening, review, or callback systems?
Tracking	Track patients?
	Track physical records?
	Track equipment and maintenance schedules?
	Track orthoses, prostheses, and implants?
Decision support	Provide clinical alerts?
	Record patient information resources?
	Provide pathway support?
	Ability to evaluate learning?
Requesting	Request diagnostic testing?
	Refer to other therapists?
	Request second opinion?
Reporting	Are there links to diagnostic test results?
	Report adverse incidents?
	Provide activity reports by variety of fields?
	Provide audit reports?
	Provide clinical effectiveness reports?
	Provide caseload and case management reports?

Table 6.1 Functions for record systems to support AHP clinical recording (*Continued*)

Function	*Does the system ... ?*
Medicines management	Allow recording of prescriptions?
	Allow recording of dispensing?
	Allow recording of medication use?
	Allow recording of medicine stock management?
Image management	Allow links to radiology reports and picture archiving and communication system (PACS) images?
	Allow recording of digital clinical images?
Document management	Save referral letters?
	Print appointments and patient contact letters?
	Print discharge letters?
	Print clinic-specific reports?
	Allow storage of legacy records?
Patient contribution area	Facilitate consent management recording?
	Allow device support, e.g. telemetry, glucose monitoring?
	Support a patient diary?
Secondary uses; audit, research, planning	Can anonymised reports be extracted for: • clinical audit • clinical governance • service management—activity and waiting times • risk management • regional and national statistics • ad hoc reporting • research?
General resource management	Resources utilisation—room and equipment?
	Alerts, e.g. stock levels?
	Staff rostering?
	Clinical supplies?
	Decontamination requirements?
	User training?
	Out-of-hours support?
Terminology	Support use of Systematised Nomenclature of Medicine (SNOMED) clinical terms?
	Support use of drug and medical devices dictionary?
	Use national data sets, data standards, and diagnostic codes?

CHAPTER 7

Using the Myers-Briggs Type Indicator within the allied health professions

Simon and Sheena Loveday

INTRODUCTION

This chapter is about the Myers-Briggs Type Indicator (MBTI),[1] a personality or 'psychometric' questionnaire widely used in business, healthcare, and personal development. The chapter sets out to explain what the MBTI is, how it can be useful to you, and how to learn more about it.

The authors of this chapter are MBTI enthusiasts and use it both inside and outside work. However, we are not setting out to seek converts. Our hope is that you will read this chapter with an open mind, but not so open that your brain falls out! By all means, be sceptical: you need to find out whether this is a method and an approach that will work for you and we welcome a readiness to challenge and question. But please, if your mind is closed already, read no further. We don't expect to convince you on the basis of one article!

The purpose of this chapter is to introduce the MBTI to AHPs and to give them an idea of how it can help us:
- to understand ourselves better
- to value ourselves and others more
- to get the best from ourselves and others
- to become more effective in our working relationships.

FIVE SCENARIOS

How might you know you're achieving these objectives? If the MBTI is the answer, what is the question? Here are five scenarios. If any of them fit—read on.

1 You have reached a decision point in your career. You have to choose between continuing in a specialist role or becoming a generalist. The financial and promotion aspects point clearly in one direction—but your instincts are set in the other. How could you get a better understanding of your reservations in this matter?

2 You work closely with a colleague. At first you really liked their quiet, thoughtful, undemonstrative style. But now it is beginning to drive you mad. The more you push for responses from them, the less you get. What can you do?

3 You are an AHP. One of your recent consultations involved a very rare complaint— you have never seen one outside a textbook. You successfully identified the problem and were successful in insisting that the patient take appropriate action. Now, to your dismay, you hear that the patient has lodged a complaint against you! What has gone wrong?

4 You work as part of a locality team. The team has agreed its targets and objectives at the start of the year and set them out clearly in a schedule—but you seem to be the only one of your colleagues who is attending to them. In previous years, your colleagues have 'got there' fine in the end, but the uncertainty and their lack of concern are driving you crazy. How can you and they come to some land of agreed style?

5 Mostly you handle work pressures pretty well—but sometimes you find yourself responding in a way that seems completely out of character. How can you prevent this happening again? And is there a way you and your colleagues can see it coming next time and either guard against it or minimise its impact?

BACKGROUND TO THE INDICATOR

The MBTI is a personality test. Its underlying principles derive from the work of Carl Jung (1875–1961),[2, 3] the brilliant Swiss psychologist and philosopher who coined, among other things, the terms 'extravert' and 'introvert'. Jung was for a number of years a close associate of Sigmund Freud, but Freud's insistence on the need for a close adherence to his beliefs and assumptions led to a breakdown of the relationship in 1911–12. This was a great shock to Jung and he spent much of the war years—Switzerland of course being neutral—trying to work out how two people could differ fundamentally and yet still 'both be right'. The result of that was *Psychological Types*. Three of the four dimensions of the indicator were set out in that book. It was translated into English in 1923 and read by an American woman with a strong interest in character and personality—Katharine Briggs—and her daughter Isabel Myers. When America entered World War II in 1942, Isabel and Katharine turned to Jung's work for two reasons: first, to find an instrument that would help people find their niche in the turmoil of conscription and war work;

and second, from a more idealistic drive closely related to Jung's, to find a way to understand and respect others, or in a phrase that became a beacon for Isabel, to 'value difference'.

The resulting questionnaire (of which there is more below) went through 30 years of research before becoming available to the general public in 1975. The research base is huge and growing and its validity has been tested and established worldwide. Over three million people take it in English each year and it is now available in 15 languages.

Before explaining what it *is*, we should explain clearly what it *isn't*. It doesn't measure ability; it doesn't measure sanity (or insanity); and it shouldn't be used (on its own at least) for selection. So what does it do?

TYPE AND PREFERENCE

The basic theories of the Indicator are built round the concepts of *type* and *prefer-ence*. The simplest way to illustrate this is to invite you to write your name—but with your wrong hand. When people describe what this is like, they tend to come up with words like 'awkward ... difficult ... takes concentration ... slow ... shaky'. Sometimes, it makes them cross—'why am I doing this when I can do it perfectly well with the other hand?'—or insecure and anxious. Sometimes, on the other hand, they find it an enjoyable challenge, even fun.

And the result? A frequent comment is that it looks 'like a child's writing'. Often people notice too that they have written very big, which in turn makes it almost exaggeratedly clear.

Doing this exercise illustrates a key way in which MBTI theory is different from most psychological theories. Most personality tests are based on a central core of normal behaviour—confidence, sociability, openness, optimism, and so on. These characteristics of personality, known as traits, are distributed along a normal dis-tribution curve: put differently, most people are in the middle. (That's why they're normal.) People with too little or too much of the trait, those who deviate from the norm, are different—or deviant. At the extremes, you don't want to employ some-one like that, and that's why personality tests can be very useful in selection.

But handwriting is different. We have a left hand and a right hand—and in the UK at least, it is perfectly valid to use either to write with. But almost everyone develops a preference, very early in life, which leads them to specialise in one or the other. We may use different hands for different things but we very seldom hesitate when it comes to picking up a pen. Either/or preferences of this kind, as opposed to 'too much/too little' theories illustrated earlier, are what psychologists mean when they talk about 'type'. And this approach has four important consequences.

1   That it's OK to have clear preferences: you can't 'prefer both'.
2   That both preferences are of equal value. Despite what some countries still teach in their schools, the left hand works just as well as the right hand.

3   That, just as you have a 'right hand', so you will have a 'wrong hand'—a less pre-
    ferred style of behaviour. And when you use that style—when shy people try to
    be more assertive, or cool and distant people try to get all warm and friendly—
    you will probably do it rather badly, at least to start with, and above all overdo it.
    That's not surprising: like your wrong-handed writing, it has been lying unused
    and undeveloped inside you for years, indeed since your childhood.

4   That you *can* do it. People may not *want* to write with their wrong hand, but eve-
    ryone can do it. With practice you would get better, to the point where perhaps
    others didn't know it was not your usual hand (though you, of course, would).
    And it might even be fun!

THE FOUR DIMENSIONS OF TYPE

Jung's theory of psychological type posits that there are a number of brain functions
that are binary, like a light switch. We can do one or the other—but we can't do
them at the same time. In this, they are like left- and right-handedness. And in the
same way, we develop a preference for one, and leave the other undeveloped.

The first of these dimensions—the E/I dimension—is about energy. People who
get their energy from the outer world of people and things, Jung called extraverts—
literally, 'turned outwards'. A preference of this kind tends to lead people to have:

* a preference for action
* a tendency to breadth, to knowing a little about a lot
* a need to do their thinking outwardly, by talking things over
* an open, 'WYSIWYG' personality—what you see is what you get!

Of course, they can do the opposite but it will drain their energy and feel like hard work.

Contrasting with them are 'introverts'. Introversion has for many years had a bad
press (there is a famous if untraceable story about a comment heard in an American
supermarket queue, 'My daughter used to be an introvert, but she's better now'). But
the term 'introversion' merely means that your energy is turned, and tuned, to the
inner world of thoughts and concepts, so that:

* you will feel most at home in your inner life
* your strengths will lie in deep reflection rather than quick action, and you will
  usually be more of a specialist, knowing 'a lot about a little' (or having few
  friends, but knowing them very well)
* you will typically keep something of yourself in reserve
* in order to give of your best, others will need to allow you time to think things
  over—to consult your inner sources of judgment and experience and to pay
  attention to what they say.

Of course, introverts can and do extrovert, but it drains their energy and can leave
them with nothing to spare for social interaction at the end of the day.

The second dimension, the S/N scale, is about how we take in information. When we use our Sensing function, we rely on the evidence from our senses—we take in what is there, what is available to our five senses. People with a well-developed preference for Sensing will tend to:
- see what is, accept reality as it is
- enjoy the material side of life
- be realistic, practical, and comfortable with detail
- adapt existing things
- focus on the past (because it is real and has really happened) and the present (because it is really happening now)
- ask 'what' question: 'What needs to be done? What do you want me to do?'

The contrasting way of taking in information is through possibilities, connections, meanings, relationships, and patterns—in essence, not seeing how things are, but how things might be. (It is sometimes said that 'scientists see what everyone has seen, but notice what nobody has noticed', and that ability to make connections and draw conclusions is characteristic of Intuition as the term is used here.) People with a well-developed preference for Intuition (it is always shortened to N to avoid confusion with I for Introversion) are likely to:
- see what might be and question reality
- be visionary, speculative, and look beyond the present and the given
- seek out 'big picture' solutions and explanations
- invent new things
- focus on the future (because it hasn't happened yet and so gives plenty of scope)
- ask 'why' questions: 'Why are we doing this? Why does it have to be like this?'

The third dimension is the T/F scale—Thinking and Feeling. This scale examines how we make decisions. Jung argued that there are two perfectly rational, but entirely separate, ways of reaching decisions. (The terms are used here in quite a special sense: 'thinkers' don't necessarily think better, and 'feelers' don't necessarily feel more.) When you use your Thinking function to make a decision, you use logical principles, you weigh things up carefully—even to the point of counting the 'for' and 'against' arguments—and you remain impersonal. If you have feelings, you seek to discount them: 'I try not to act according to feelings unless there is a rational explanation for them' (Thinking type quoted in Bayne, 1995). Thinking seeks to fit the world, and our experiences, into a logical order. And its ultimate goal—even if there is a price to pay for it—is truth.

The Feeling function reaches decisions differently—with reference to values and beliefs. What is the most important value at stake in a decision? What is the right thing to do? Your guide is values and beliefs—sometimes accessed almost by instinct rather than by a process that you can spell out and make explicit. The Feeling function emphasises relationship and connection (rather than the detachment that is a key value for the Thinking function). Feeling seeks to fit the world, and our experiences, into a moral order. And the prime goal of feeling—even if there is a price to pay for it—is harmony.

The three dimensions that we have looked at so far are those that Jung himself identified in *Psychological Types*. But Isabel and Katharine added a fourth, based on earlier research by Katharine. This is the J/P scale—Judging and Perceiving—and it identifies how we like to live our outer lives. (This, incidentally, is the scale that often plays out most visibly in family life!) People with a Judging preference seek closure; they wish their lives were organised, planned, and controlled, they like the comfort of getting things decided and settled, and they enjoy having dates in the diary so that they know where they will be and what they will be doing well into the future, thus minimising uncertainty. Not surprisingly, a lot of Js are managers in organisations: after all, they like things to be organised! They are usually great list-makers—not just making lists, but enjoying the sensuous pleasure of crossing things off them as they get done. If you want to keep a Judging type happy, remember their motto: No surprises!

People with a Perceiving preference look across at Judging types and think … how sad! Get a life! The Perceiving preference is for incoming information—for leaving things open as long as possible—for curiosity, spontaneity, variety, and trying things out to see if you like them. (Tigger's exploratory approach to diet in *Winnie the Pooh* is a perfect example of Perceiving in action.) Judging types can make themselves adapt; Perceiving types naturally prefer adaptability and flexibility. The structure that gives Judging types confidence and security is experienced by Perceiving types as a constraint and a prison: Don't tie me down! And the readiness of Perceiving types to leave things to the last minute—because that's the only way it is possible to guarantee having the maximum amount of information—is seen by Judging types as disorganisation and procrastination.

The linkages with family life are most obvious here: Perceiving children leaving their homework to the last minute, to the dismay of their Judging parents; the Judging partner wanting their week—or their holiday—carefully structured with every day filled, while the Perceiving partner wants to leave things open and 'see how I feel on the day'; the Judging partner sustained by lists, the Perceiving partner watching with puzzled amusement.

How do these four preferences play out in the daily reality of work and home life? The first thing to say is that they are preferences, not rigid rules: we all use all the behavioural styles, and indeed the ability to work outside our preferred style is a mark of maturity and the fully developed personality. But to be able to use a less preferred style is not the same as preferring that style. Our preferred style is like our home—it's where we feel safe and comfortable. We don't spend all our time there, but we need to know where it is.

The second point to make is that these preferences don't work in isolation. Like ingredients in a menu, they work together to produce a whole person. There are

16 possible combinations of the four letters. If we take four at random—Introversion, Sensing, Thinking, and Judging—we come up with the ISTJ type.
- Introversion provides reflection and depth.
- Sensing provides realism and an eye for detail.
- Thinking provides logic and firmness.
- Judging provides organisation and follow-through.

If we look at the polar opposite, ENFP, we see the contrasting preferences.
- Extraversion providing breadth and a need for human contact.
- Intuition providing vision and a grasp of possibilities.
- Feeling providing warmth and empathy.
- Perceiving providing flexibility and adaptability.

The theory predicts that the sober, sensible ISTJs will be overrepresented in managerial positions—organisers love organisations!—and the statistics support this. Conversely, the theory would lead us to expect that in organisations, the sociable, optimistic ENFP types are usually found in the marketing department—and they are!

Finally, the type description can be uncannily accurate. If we take the short description in Jenny Rogers' manual,[4] we find:

> Thoughtful, responsible and perfectionist, ISTJs need to be in charge. This can be both an asset and a liability, depending on how it is linked to the ISTJ's skills and experience'.

Many readers will recognise a colleague—and perhaps themselves! But there is more. The MBTI can illustrate behaviour in a wide range of different contexts—leadership, team membership, ideal organisation, relationships, and change. It can predict behaviour under stress. And—perhaps most usefully—it can offer a list of ways to become more effective. All these are concentrated onto a single page in the Rogers manual.

So let us look at our five scenarios and see how type might cast light on them. The first was individual:

You have reached a decision point in your career. You have to choose between continuing in a specialist role or becoming a generalist. The financial and promotion aspects point clearly in one direction—but your instincts are set in the other. How could you get a better understanding of your reservations in this matter?

We have seen that type descriptions can give you a very full account of your preferences for the land of environment—for colleagues, for type of work, for leadership—that will get the best from you at work. But we can go a little further than this. The theory predicts that each type will have a dominant function—an overriding goal in life. To take our ISTJ example, type theory would predict that to be fulfilled in their work, this person would need:

To notice and work on something useful to others, quietly, systematically, and in-depth.[5]

And contrastingly, ENFPs will need 'to find lots of new and stimulating possibilities and promote new ventures'. A lens of this nature turned onto a job can be very revealing. Can the job ever satisfy the basic drive that gets you out of bed in the morning? This kind of insight can help you tell the difference between the natural prudence and caution that anyone might feel before a challenging and demanding change of direction—and a real sense that you are about to take an irreversible wrong turn.

The second was about a clash of working styles with a colleague:

You work closely with a colleague. At first you really liked their quiet, thoughtful, and undemonstrative style. But now it is beginning to drive you mad. The more you push for responses from them, the less you get. What can you do?

The more you seek a response, the less response you get. Of course, there may be many reasons for this, but a good place to start is with the Extraversion/Introversion scale. Extraverts need stimulus and response from the outside world, and they formulate their thoughts by talking them over aloud. (How do I know what I think, until I see what I say?) If your preference is for Extraversion, then the Introvert's quiet internal processing of ideas—'I think over what I'm going to say, and then I realise that having done that, there's no need to say it'—is a constant frustration to you: what are they thinking? How can I do my thinking, with nothing to respond to? Now look at it from the Introvert's side. The more the Extravert talks, the less you can think; just when you are ready to start talking—the Extravert jumps in and fills the silence. No wonder you don't say much!

Below is a list of ways Extraverts and Introverts can communicate better. If your colleague prefers Introversion—or is using an Introvert style with you—then try:

- giving them thinking time
- giving them information in writing where possible
- waiting for a response, so that they have time to 'mull things over'
- checking things out rather than taking silence for agreement.

But communication is a two-way street. How can your quiet, reserved colleague get the best out of you? By:

- letting you talk things over
- telling you things in person, rather than in writing/by e-mail
- giving you space for action and experiment
- allowing you to develop your thoughts as you talk, without assuming that the first thoughts should be the final conclusions.

But there is something that underlies these actions you can take. It is a change of attitude: a question, to use an earlier phrase, of 'valuing difference'. Introverts aren't just quiet extraverts; extraverts aren't just noisy introverts. Each is actually using a different process—and if you start by respecting that and allowing it to work in its way, rather than yours, you're likely to get a much better result.

Now for our third scenario. (A recent Radio Four programme claimed that one-third of complaints from patients about GPs were about 'poor communication'.)

You are a GP. One of your recent consultations involved a very rare complaint—you have never seen one outside a textbook. You successfully identified the problem and managed, despite the patient's initial resistance, to persuade them to take appropriate action. Now, to your dismay, you hear that the patient has lodged a complaint against you! What has gone wrong?

The question of the match of communication styles between patients and GPs has been the subject of much attention in recent years. Research shows that the most common preferences in doctors are N and T (Intuition and Thinking), while the most common preferences in the population at large are Sensing and Feeling.[6] How does each group like to communicate? Research indicates that there is what we might call a 'language problem'.

People with N and T—big ideas and logic—naturally talk a particular 'language': theoretical, concise, minimal, stripped of detail, focused on the task and the problem. If they want to work with another person, they need to respect them first (if necessary by challenging them to establish that they are truly competent)—then they can build a relationship. And that is of course perfectly suited to much of the technical work of diagnosis and treatment.

But people with S and F—sometimes called 'sensible and friendly' for short—have a different communication style: practical, extended, thorough, wanting every T crossed and every I dotted, and needing to focus on the person behind the problem. For SFs, the relationship is the starting point—if they can build that, then they are willing to trust the other person's competence.

To quote a recent research study:

> If you are a patient with preferences for Sensing with Feeling (40.1% of the UK population), then you will have only a one in six chance of seeing a doctor with the same preferences. Similarly, if you are a doctor with preferences for Intuition and Thinking (31.3% of this sample), you will have only a one in 11 chance that your patient will be the same as you. Some adjustment on the part of one or both parties involved in the interaction is, therefore, likely to be needed if effective communication is to occur. These results may contribute, therefore, to the explanation of the number of complaints from patients about poor communication, the lack of understanding, and poor compliance reported in the literature if these doctors have not learned to adjust their interaction styles to accommodate these differences.[6]

So what happened in the consulting room? Well, one hypothesis is that this is a case of a breakdown in communication between NT and SF styles. To the NT doctor, the successful outcome is a diagnosis and a treatment. To the SF patient, something has gone wrong in the relationship: perhaps they have been seen as a disease rather than as a person; they haven't been treated as a human being; they haven't been recognised as an individual. Neither side is right, but something must be done to bridge the gap—and knowing something about the other person's 'language' is an essential starting point.

Our fourth scenario was about teamwork:

You work as part of a practice team. The team has agreed on its targets and objectives at the start of the year and set them out clearly in a schedule—but you seem to be the only one of your colleagues who is attending to them. In previous years, your colleagues have 'got there' fine in the end, but the uncertainty and their lack of concern are driving you crazy. How can you and they come to some kind of agreed style?

By now you will recognise that the mismatch here is likely to be along the J/P dimension. The person with the Judging preference makes lists and plans in the expectation that they will be used as roadmaps and reference points throughout the year: that targets and objectives are not just aiming marks, but real destinations that you intend to arrive at. It looks as though they are surrounded by Perceiving types—whose attention is on the changing world around them, and whose focus is not on what was planned to be done months ago, but on what needs to be done right now. If you are indeed a J and they are indeed Ps—how can you find a way to not be driven crazy?

There is a clue in the penultimate sentence of the scenario. Your colleagues do get there in the end. Their way does work—but it fills you with anxiety (just as yours probably fill them with impatience!). If both of you are willing to respect the other's style as something that works, however strange it is to you, then here are some ways to bridge the style gap. To get the best from your Perceiving colleagues, you need to recognise that your structures and lists are not their favourite thing, so you need to:

• show you are flexible
• leave space for them to surprise you
• be prepared to change your mind.

And on their side? To come half way to meet you and respect your discomfort with the unstructured and unplanned, it will probably help you greatly if they would be willing to:

• show they are organised
• give you some kind of plan or indication of how their work is developing
• allow you to complain and 'tut tut' without being too discomposed!

Our final scenario is about stress—a topic much to the fore in the healthcare literature.

Mostly you handle work pressures pretty well—but sometimes you find yourself responding in a way that seems completely out of character. How can you prevent this happening again? And is there a way you and your colleagues can see it coming next time, and either guard against it, or minimise its impact?

For this topic, we need to go back to the 'wrong hand' exercise. Jungian theory, and Myers-Briggs likewise, emphasise that it isn't possible to be perfect—that you will always have preferences and develop aspects of yourself to different levels, so that some parts of you remain less developed than others. When you are able to use your preferred style, then work pressure is challenging and exciting. When you are pushed into using those less preferred sides, you feel stressed, and all the consequences of that come into play, just as we saw in the 'wrong hand' exercise at the start of this chapter. How the MBTI can help is to explain where your 'wrong hand' is and how stress will affect you. If you know your four-letter type, you know what stresses that type, and you know how that type responds to stress. And if you know it, you can use that information in three ways. First, you can guard against the situations that cause you stress. Second, you can learn to recognise the symptoms and take appropriate action. And finally, you can enlist the help of your colleagues. The more they know about your strengths and weaknesses—and vice versa—the better able they are to cover for you, to recognise what is happening to you, and to find appropriate ways of dealing with the consequences.

HOW DO YOU TAKE IT FORWARD?

- You can read more about it—there is a short reading list at the end of this chapter.
- You can arrange to take the Indicator yourself. For this, you need the services of a trained and qualified MBTI practitioner, because it is a skilled process to help someone to find their type. Like an experienced tailor or dressmaker, the practitioner will help you try the suit for size and 'find the fit'—the questionnaire results are not the final arbiter, and it is a core principle of the MBTI that 'the person taking the test is the best judge of their type'. Most parts of the NHS have qualified practitioners, or the national MBTI body, the British Association for Psychological Type (www.bapt.org.uk), will provide names of practitioners in your area.
- You can go to BAPT meetings to learn more about the instrument—this chapter has only scratched the surface of its many applications. It provides sessions for qualified practitioners, but also for those with more curiosity than experience. BAPT details are given in the bibliography.
- You can explore how to get qualified—one of the joys of the Indicator is that it is possible to be qualified without being a trained psychologist. In the UK, Oxford Psychologists Press (www.opp.co.uk) has acquired a training monopoly, but in America and Australia there are a number of excellent training providers. A Google search under 'MBTI qualifying' is all you need. Surprisingly, it is cheaper to fly to Florida and qualify with CAPT (www.capt.org) than it is to qualify in the UK—and you could even take the family to Disney World while you're there!

REFERENCES

1. Myers P, Briggs I. *Gifts Differing.* Palo Alto, CA: Consulting Psychologists Press; 1980.
2. Jung CG. *Psychological Types.* London: Routledge; 1923.
3. Jung CG. A psychological theory of types. In: *Modern Man in Search of a Soul.* London: Routledge; 1933, reprinted 1978.
4. Rogers J. *Sixteen Personality Types at Work in Organisations.* London: Management Futures Ltd; 1997.
5. Bayne R. *The Myers-Briggs Type Indicator: a critical review and practical guide.* London: Chapman and Hall; 1995.
6. Clack GB. *Personality Differences Between Doctors and Their Patients: implications for the teaching of communication skills.* Unpublished research; 2003.

FURTHER READING

Further reading and information (chosen from a huge list of articles and books).

- Allen, J, Brock S. *Healthcare Communication: using personality type.* London: Routledge 2001. (How MBTI can illuminate the way patients and health professionals relate to each other, well provided with examples and anecdotes.)
- Allen J, Houghton A. Understanding personality type. *BMJ.* 2005; 330: 35–7.
- Baron R. *What Type am I? Discover who you really are.* New York: Penguin; 1998.
- British Association for Psychological Type (BAPT). Available at: www.bapt.org. uk. (BAPT is the Myers-Briggs user group and provides information and events to publicise the instrument and bring users and potential users together.)
- Hammer AL. *Introduction to Type and Careers.* Palo Alto, CA: Consulting Psychologists Press; 1998.
- Houghton A. Extraversion and introversion, a series of short articles about the MBTI published in the *British Medical Journal,* which can also be found on their website, http://careerfocus.bmjjournals.com. 2004; 329: 191–2).
- (2004; 329: 202–3) How do you like to take in information?
- (2004; 329: 213–14) How do you make decisions? Thinking and feeling.
- (2004; 329: 230–31) How do you like to live your life? Judging and perceiving.
- (2004; 329: 241–2) The whole type and how it relates to job satisfaction.
- (2005; 329: 8–9) What do type dynamics tell us about life stages and stress reactions? (2005; 330: 18–19) Type and teams.

CHAPTER 8

Appraisal: 360° feedback

Simon and Sheena Loveday

When we were asked to write this chapter, our first reaction was, 'Why us?' The reason was a session one of us had given on this topic at an NHS leadership-training event. The person who put us forward for this chapter had been a participant on the programme. She had come into the session feeling, 'I couldn't possibly do this—much too scary'. She left feeling, 'This feels well worthwhile—and I think I could do it'. If readers of this chapter leave with the same feeling, then our time in writing it will have been well spent.

INTRODUCTION: WHAT IS 360° FEEDBACK? AND WHAT IS THE POINT OF GATHERING IT?

360° feedback is simply a method for gathering information from those around you about the effectiveness of your behaviour. 'Feedback' refers to a response or reaction; '360°' indicates that it goes right round the compass to cover all angles on you and what you do, from your boss above you, through your peers beside you, to your reports below you in the organisational tree. When you set out to gather 360° feedback, you are simply asking those most affected by your behaviour to tell you how your behaviour impacts upon them, what messages (intentional or unintentional) you are sending, what works well—and what needs improving.

Put as simply as that, it is perhaps strange that we don't use the technique more often. After all, we interact with others every day, and our behaviour affects them constantly. The same is true in reverse: others' behaviour affects us all the time, and sometimes we long for the opportunity to encourage them to do more of what works—or to find ways to stop them doing what doesn't work. Organisations use it a lot in the form of questionnaires and satisfaction surveys; car manufacturers, garages, supermarkets, hotels, local councils, and even training providers are constantly asking us whether we are happy with what they do. Feedback—in the sense we are using here—is now a fact of life. And given that our behaviour is the only tool we have for influencing others, it would be strange if we didn't invest some serious time in finding out whether the tool is working properly.

However, most of us also have a degree of apprehension in asking others for feedback—particularly such 'significant others' as bosses, peers, reports, and customers (or patients). One apprehension is about the possibility of 'bad news'— what if they don't like the way we behave toward them? Worse, what if they don't like who we are? How will we face them at work when we know that?

Curiously, however, another apprehension is about good news. The English reluctance to confront feelings directly means that direct praise can be as embarrassing as direct criticism. So even getting good feedback and enthusiastic affirmation of what we do can still be uncomfortable!

How might we overcome this reluctance?

A good way, we would suggest, is to reframe the whole concept of 360° feedback. Its parenthood is stern. Its father is appraisal—a manager assessing and judging the effectiveness of the work of a member of their staff. Its mother, born perhaps 30 years ago, is upward appraisal—direct reports assessing and judging the effectiveness of the person who manages them. But 360° feedback at its best is different from both its parents. This difference is best thought of in three ways.

- As a process, not the one-off annual event of appraisal.
- To remember that it is about development, not about assessment. Apart from your boss, those whom you ask for feedback won't have power over you or over your salary.
- This one grows from the first two—not as a method of judging your effectiveness, but rather as a way of involving others in your development. Used correctly, 360° feedback gives others the chance to help you be more effective, to grow, and to develop. And most of your respondents will be pleased to be asked—and appreciative of the chance to be involved in this process.

SO WHY USE THIS PROCESS?

The most important question is the initial one: Why do you want feedback? What do you want feedback about?

There can be a variety of reasons. Perhaps you are going for a promotion, or for a development opportunity such as a leadership workshop, and want to check out your performance in your current role. Perhaps you lead a team and want to hear both from them and from your boss what you do that works and what you could do better. Perhaps you want to involve customers, peers, service users, or patients in the process. Perhaps you are unsure of what your strengths are. Perhaps you are very well aware of some aspects of your behaviour that get in the way—but you are working on them and want to know if those aspects are still a problem. Perhaps you have never looked in the mirror in this way before, and feel that it is time you did a reality check. And perhaps you feel that it is important to consult others because they are on the receiving end of what you do and you want to show them that you take their views seriously.

The great benefit of the 360° process is the reality check—the ability to 'see ourselves as others see us'. But it is not without its risks. One risk is outside you—that some of the recipients might use it as an opportunity to offload on you grudges and grievances that are not really yours at all, but belong to the organisation. Another 'outside' risk is that people will tell you what they think you want to hear. But the principle risk is inside you—that you will hear something that you are unable or unwilling to receive. If you don't want, or don't feel strong enough, or don't feel ready, to hear others' views, the answer is simple: don't ask. Don't embark on the process until you feel ready to take it on.

So, as in most things, there can be 'enemies without' and 'enemies within'. How can we tackle these?

First, it is helpful to ask yourself, 'Is there anything about me, or the way I receive comments, that could make people reluctant to be honest with me? Am I very sensitive to criticism? How ready will others be to speak their minds?' Second, it is well to ask yourself how your manager will respond: will their comments be constructive, or will they just take it as an opportunity to dwell on any weaknesses they see? And third, think about the context around you. Is now the right moment for the exercise? Will your respondents give it their full attention? Will they see it for what it is, or will they find some sinister ulterior motive in it? Is the organisation one in which it is possible for staff and colleagues to speak honestly and directly? Again, if you're not sure of the answers to these questions, you need to explore further before you launch in.

PUTTING IT INTO PRACTICE: CHOOSING THE RIGHT METHOD

The first question is always, 'What sort of data do you want?' That will always determine the kind of questions you ask. You might want to know how you perform against a set of competencies (e.g., the Leadership Qualities Framework, or a more general leadership or managerial competency framework). You might want to know what you need to do in order to maximise your chances of promotion. You might want to know how you're doing as a team leader—as a team member—as a colleague—as an AHP practitioner. You might simply be interested in your own development for its own sake.

When you start to look at the range of 360° tools and instruments on the market, you will be amazed. (A recent search on Google had 34 900 results.) There are huge numbers, and great complexity. A good selection principle is to remember when you filled in a feedback form for someone else. How easy was it? How quick?

How satisfying? At the end, did you feel you had said what you wanted to say, or were your answers cramped and constrained by the format of the questions? There are a number of questionnaires that look impressive in their range and numerical thoroughness, but that suffer from two problems. The first is 'respondent fatigue'— which sets in relatively quickly! And the second is spurious precision. A lot of questionnaires ask for number scores and will add, average, and differentiate them in clever ways, but it is difficult to know what weight to put on the original scores. If you ask to be rated on a 1–5 scale, someone with low expectations may rate you at 5 because you are better than they expected. Someone else may rate you at only 4 because they never give 5s. And a third respondent may rate you at only 2 because they are fed up with managers (or team leaders, or consultants, or whatever category you fall into) and all they want is an excuse to work off their frustration. How do you add up these incompatible ratings and get a meaningful average? So be wary of complexity for its own sake.

A good rule of thumb is:

- ask only the questions that matter to you in your current situation
- ask both for numbers and for comments (quantitative and qualitative data)
- stick to words that will have meaning for your respondents
- end with an open-ended question
- and above all: keep it short!

HOW TO GATHER THE FEEDBACK

You have a number of choices. Do you want the comments to be made in writing, or given to you face-to-face? (A good combination is to use both: ask people to complete a questionnaire, then talk it through with you. For more on this, see 'Receiving the feedback' below.)

If in writing, do you want hard copy or e-mail? E-mail is quick and easy and people like it; the response rate is usually better. But some of your respondents may not have access to it, and there may be security or confidentiality issues.

If entirely face-to-face without anything in writing, you must take notes and, very importantly, you must check them back with the respondent at the end of the session to ensure that what you heard is really what they said.

You may feel that the people—or the culture—aren't ready for the openness of direct feedback, and that you will get a better and more honest response if you ask for anonymous comments so that respondents feel more free to speak their minds—and so that you feel more confidence in positive comments. And since it will be difficult for respondents to maintain that anonymity if comments come directly to you (you'll often recognise handwriting, and it's hard to send an anonymous e-mail!), then you can ask a third party to collect and collate comments for you. This of course is where external providers come in. If you go to an external provider, make sure that you look at a sample profile to see how they treat the data. Two questions worth asking are, do they include all the raw data? (They should. It's the most powerful part.) And do they summarise the salient points for you—and if so, how? (Be sceptical of so-called 'intelligent systems' that produce text reports. Systems they may be, but they aren't always very intelligent.)

Don't just ask others for their scores and comments—enter yours on the questionnaire as well. (If nothing else, it will tell you whether the questionnaire is easy and practical to complete, or the reverse.) Self-assessment is interesting for its own sake, but its primary value is to give you a reference point when you're reading respondents' scores and comments. If you think you're weak in a certain area and they do too, then at least your reality matches theirs. If your views and theirs don't match, you've learned something worth knowing—and better still, something worth investigating.

Further points to look out for in questionnaire design? On the numerical side, our experience is that a scale of 1–5 is best; ensure that people know whether 1 is low or high (mark it on every page). Give respondents the option of leaving a blank or ticking a 'don't know' box if they want to—otherwise you will not be able to tell whether a 3 is a genuine middle score or a way of saying that there is not enough evidence either way.

WHAT QUESTIONS TO ASK

As usual, it depends on what answers you want! We can split this into four possibilities. The first is to use a standard 360° questionnaire, either one current in your organisation, or a commercially available one. This has the advantage of saving you a lot of work; it will probably be quite thorough and wide-ranging; and it may give you some useful comparative data against a benchmark of other organisations. On the downside, it may not ask quite the questions you want answered, it won't use precisely the language of your organisation—and you may have to pay for it.

A second option, if your organisation has a list of competencies that are applicable to your role, is to simply send around that list and ask people to rate you against each competency on a 1–5 scale. That is again quite labour-saving (for you), it is specific to your organisation, and it is respectful of the fact that the organisation has put time and money into developing the competencies. The biggest disadvantages are, first, that there are sometimes quite a lot of competencies—and second, that many competencies appear only distantly related to the real world of work, with the result that respondents don't find it very easy to write genuine answers that express what they want to say. Of how many of your colleagues could you say that they:

Accurately interpret the underlying causes of others' behaviour, recognising their needs, concerns, and feelings whether expressed or implicit?

Would you want to rate a colleague for:

> Understands and conveys the mission and vision of the organisation with passion and conviction?

(Indeed, would you want to work with anyone like that?) The Leadership Qualities Framework is not always beyond reproach here.

If it is your leadership qualities and potential that you want to explore, you might try the approach suggested by Pedler and Burgoyne in their *Manager's Guide to Self-Development*. They put forward seven criteria for effective leadership—and offer a simple questionnaire that asks respondents not only to rate you, but to rate the importance of each quality. You may not find the seven criteria completely convincing but what the method does provide is a simple grid that enables you to identify at a glance the areas where your respondents feel you need to focus.

A third option, as we have seen, is to design your own questionnaire focusing on what you want to find out. An elegant preliminary to this is to ask your respondents—your patients, for example, or the members of your team—what qualities are important to them, what they are looking for from you, and then to use these questions so that they have in effect designed the questionnaire that they will then be asked to respond to. This method has a lot to recommend it!

With all three methods, it depends on how much information you want. (That's one reason why it's a good idea to fill out the questionnaire yourself before you give it to others.) If you want a lot of information, encourage your respondents to provide examples by every question. But whatever method you use, it's always a good idea to provide an opportunity for participants to write what they want to say—rather than what you want to ask. A simple and well-proven way to do this is to use the A4 page suggested below (*see* Box 8.1): the page can go either at the start or the finish of the questionnaire.

Box 8.1 Preliminary questionnaire

Pen Picture: what words or phrases would you use to describe this person?
What do you see as their special strengths? What qualities do they bring to their job?
(Optional, if you are exploring your further career development) How do you see their future in your organisation?
In order to be at their most effective, is there anything they should do differently?

We suggested that there were four options. The fourth option is simply to use the page above on its own. It is quick and easy for respondents to complete and for you or your data-collector to process; and its simplicity not only increases the likelihood of a response, but also ensures that the big issues will leap off the page. Moreover, they will be phrased in the respondents' own words. Those are not inconsiderable advantages!

WHO (AND HOW MANY) TO ASK

The first and best rule is, 'Ask people whose opinions you respect'. If you aren't going to listen to the answer, don't bother to ask the question. By definition, 360° feedback has some givens in it: upwards, sideways, and downwards. But there is often some choice in that. If you do have a choice, don't feel that you have to 'seek balance' by going out of your way to include someone who you know dislikes you or has a low opinion of you. That isn't balance. That's tokenism, and it allows you to say, 'I know where that comment comes from—and I don't have to pay attention to it because they always say that about me'. Go for people you can learn from: people you respect, and who know you well enough for their opinions and judgments to matter to you. They may or may not dislike you or be in conflict with you; what matters is that you value what they say. And it doesn't have to be people who have known you a long time. It can equally be people who haven't been in your team or your work environment for long, so that what you are learning is how you come across at the first impression.

A good second rule is to look at your important relationships—the ones that repay an investment of time and energy. That may include clients or key internal customers; it may also include your secretary or PA.

Don't be put off by closeness. By all means, ask work colleagues who are also friends (as long as you know that friendship won't get in the way of honesty). If it's a personal topic you're interested in, feel free to ask friends outside work, and even partners or close family. But don't only ask the people you get on with. Be prepared to ask those you don't get on with too. Just stick to the two basic rules above: important relationships and opinions you will respect.

A final point about numbers. A lot of the commercial questionnaires advise you to ask widely—up to 12 or 14 people. Part of the reason is because they assume there will be a wide dropout rate, but there is also an assumption that more data mean a better result. We would challenge that assumption. In our view, this exercise is about finding the key points that you need to work on in order to be more effective—and more information is as likely to confuse the issue as it is to clarify it. We would suggest six to eight is an ideal number—and aim for at least an 80% return rate. Which brings us to briefing.

BRIEFING YOUR RESPONDENTS

A good starting point, once again, is to think of yourself as a respondent. Which will motivate you more, make you feel more important and valued—and increase the likelihood of your giving quality feedback: a visit from a colleague to ask for your help and explain the reasons or an e-mail with an attachment? Most people respond better to the first, and that is the method we will advocate here. If you are going to brief your respondents, it's probably worth booking a few minutes with them—the middle of a busy office is not a good place—and ensuring that you can find a place where you can both talk freely and without disturbance. The process need not take long, but will probably need to cover:

- explaining why you are seeking feedback at all
- explaining why you have chosen that particular person
- giving them permission to speak freely (asking for some balance between support and challenge is a good way to do this)
- explaining the sequence of events and what is expected of them (Is it anonymous? Who do they return the form to? How will it be processed? And how soon?)
- clarifying the timescale
- asking for any questions or uncertainties on their part.

Finally, and most importantly:
- thanking them in advance for their help.

It is perfectly possible to put all this in a letter, e-mail, or phone call, but face-to-face works best and sends out the message that you value the person and have chosen them personally.

USING OTHER INSTRUMENTS

One of the ways you can help respondents to give you good feedback is to identify the points that give you concern. Are you worried that you might be a bit too pushy? Not pushy enough? Over-concerned with detail? Not sufficiently concerned with detail? The answer is simply to ask: 'I'd particularly like feedback on whether I've got the right balance with detail/firmness/pace'—or whatever your concern is.

This process can be sharpened and focused by the use of personality questionnaires. Most questionnaires give you a view of what you are like at your best—and what you are like at your worst! The one we will touch on here is the Belbin team role questionnaire, which is available at www.belbin.com for a modest fee. R Meredith Belbin, an occupational psychologist, designed this questionnaire in the 1980s as result of research carried out at Henley Management College. He and his research colleagues identified eight team roles (since expanded to nine) that are essential if a team is to function properly. All of us will have a preference for a particular team role. Belbin's descriptions identify for each team role a key contribution that people with that preference bring to the team—but also what he delightfully calls an 'allowable weakness', which is, of course, the same strength,

Table 8.1 Belbin Shaper role

Strength (key quality they bring to the team)	Allowable weakness (how they may irritate other team members)
Shaper	
Dynamic, outgoing, competitive. Challenges, pressurises, finds ways round obstacles. Drives team to finish first.	Prone to impatience (which may or may not be successfully contained!).

but overdone. A good example is what he calls the Shaper role—the tough, driving leader who helps the team to strive for excellence, and without whom the team too easily settles for second best. Table 8.1 shows what Belbin says about the Shaper role.

If you take the questionnaire and find out that your preferred role is indeed Shaper, then you can easily add that description to your briefing, asking whether your respondents see either positive or negative signs of that characteristic in you—and whether the negative side is a concern to them. (Remember that they may well see the weakness, but be prepared to put up with it on the grounds that the benefits outweigh the costs. It is, after all, in Belbin's term, 'allowable'!)

A general principle of any exercise of this type is that when personality characteristics are openly acknowledged, they are much easier to deal with. Perfection isn't given to many human beings: honesty is.

RECEIVING THE FEEDBACK

So you have decided an area to explore, selected a method, and chosen and briefed your respondents. How will you go about receiving the feedback?

Receiving written feedback

Most feedback is received in writing—either 'raw' or summarised into a report. The first thing to say is that feedback about ourselves is amazingly difficult to hear and take in clearly. It is sometimes said that feedback is like a torch: when we point it at others, we see them more clearly, but when it is pointed at us, it blinds us and prevents us from seeing anything at all. So don't expect to absorb it all at once: sleep on it first.

A good way to come back to it and process it is to write a little grid that looks like Figure 8.1, using two axes: expected/unexpected, and positive/negative (or corrective). (There are other ways to do this, but this will do for now.)

These four boxes can tell you a great deal. Is there nothing much in any of the boxes? Perhaps your respondents don't feel confident (or involved) enough to give you much feedback. Is there a lot in the top two boxes? (Remember to have a look at your self-assessments to see what you wrote about yourself before you heard others'

1 Unexpected corrective feedback	2 Unexpected positive feedback
3 Expected corrective feedback	4 Expected positive feedback

Figure 8.1 Feedback grid

views.) If there is, then your self-image doesn't entirely match reality. Is there a lot in Box 4? Then you have had some useful confirmation that you are on the right track. Or is there a lot in Box 1? Then you really do have some work to do—and some conversations to have.

The final part of this written dialogue with yourself is to complete a final box (*see* Box 8.2).

Box 8.2 Self-dialogue
Areas I need to develop
Actions I need to take
People I need to talk to

RECEIVING FEEDBACK—OR CHECKING IT OUT—FACE-TO-FACE

It may be that you have the opportunity to talk through some of your feedback face-to-face. We started this chapter by suggesting that:

360° feedback is simply a method for gathering information from those around you about the effectiveness of your behaviour.

That is a good frame of mind in which to approach a face-to-face session, whether it is new information, or checking out what you have already heard: an attitude of detached curiosity, in which both giver and receiver are engaged in a joint project. Some points here are obvious: set aside enough time—up to an hour if possible; find a quiet place; keep an open mind; and take notes. Some are less obvious. One is, always ask for evidence:

You say I'm very effective as a leader. What is it that I do that makes you say that? Where have you seen me be effective?
You say that I'm not always sensitive to others' needs and feelings. What is it that I do that makes you say that? Where have you seen this happen?

A second way of drawing out information is to use the formula, 'and is there anything else?'

Third, give permission to your respondent to speak openly—not just by explicitly inviting open feedback, but also by offering specific ways into that feedback:

I've had comments that I can be a bit short-tempered and that's something I'd particularly like to check out.

I am working on being simpler and clearer and I'd like your views on whether that's succeeding.

People with my Myers-Briggs Type Indicator (MBTI) can find it a bit difficult to share their thinking with others, and I'd like to find out whether that's causing a problem.

Fourth, remember that you're on the same side as your respondent: what they're giving you is what you've asked for, so don't interrupt, contradict, or try to justify yourself or your behaviour. (We denned feedback earlier as 'a way of involving others in your development'.) You don't have to act on what they say—but the least you can do is to hear it, explore it, and take note of it. How you receive feedback will determine whether you go on getting it!

So, end by thanking them and by asking them if you can come back to them with any questions later. Very few people will say no.

SO WHAT NEXT—HOW DO YOU FOLLOW UP?

We suggested in a previous section that you would do well to list the areas you need to develop, the actions you need to take, and—crucially—the people you need to talk to. If the exercise has been worth undertaking, it is surely worth sharing the results with your manager (given that they were involved anyway). One action you will certainly want to carry out is to thank those who responded to your request; one action you might want to take is to share with them the key points from your feedback and the actions you are taking as a result. You might ask respondents if they are willing to give you continuing help with your development points:

I'm working on this area and would like to know how I'm doing … if you see me do this, please tell me.

REFERENCES

1. Pedler, J. Burgoyne M. *Managers Guide to Self-Development*. London: McGrawHill 1998/2001.
2. The Belbin Questionnaire. Available online: www.belbin.com
3. Belbin RM. *Management Teams: why they succeed* or fail.Oxford: Heinneman.1981.

CHAPTER 9

Four basic behavioural styles

Anne Mandy and Gail Louw

INTRODUCTION

A person's behavioural style exists from childhood and is a function of both heredity and environment. Each person has a dominant behavioural style that is reflected in how that individual works, interacts, and communicates with others. This behavioural style is readily observed by others, but is often difficult to identify correctly in oneself. Therefore, the development of observation skills and the application of these to an individual is the key to understanding a person's behavioural style. Similarly, the best way to identify one's own behavioural style is to receive knowledgeable and insightful feedback from others.

Bolton and Bolton[1] suggest that there are four categories of behavioural style described in Box 9.1.

1　The analyser.
2　The director.
3　The socialiser.
4　The relater.

Box 9.1 Categories of behavioural style
- **The analyser—the thought person**
  This behavioural style incorporates a low level of assertiveness and a low level of responsiveness. Analysers exhibit behaviours that are precise, deliberate, and systematic. They assimilate and process information without emotion. Such an approach results in information being gathered and evaluated prior to it being articulated or actioned. Such people are generally industrious, objective, and well-organised but rarely combine work with friendship

---

or express feelings of warmth. In addition, analysers exhibit traits of self-control and caution and are considered to be people who prefer analytical justification to emotional claims. As a result of this, they are often viewed as being a bit formal and tend to resist compromise in problem situations.

- **The director—the action person**
  This style combines a low level of emotional responsiveness with a relatively high degree of assertiveness. Such individuals tend to be task-oriented, are focused, able to express themselves succinctly, and get to the point quickly. Directors are independent and demonstrate behaviours that are often pragmatic, results-oriented, objective, and competitive. They are achievers and are commonly found in positions of authority and are central to decision-making processes in organisations. Directors are firm and forceful people, and they are confident, decisive, and generally risk-takers in interactive situations. Such traits are often perceived as concerning for colleagues, which in turn can result in conflict. Moreover, the directors leave little doubt about who is in charge of an issue that is being considered.

- **The socialiser—the front man**
  This behavioural style integrates high levels of both emotional responsiveness and assertiveness. Such people are creative and inspirational and are able to take an overview from a different perspective. They employ novel and creative approaches to problems and are willing to take risks in order to seize opportunities, particularly in interactive situations. They therefore act quickly and make instant decisions. They have a developed ability to charm, persuade, enthuse, and motivate people and can be a strong motivating force. They may be perceived as radical, extraverted, and overzealous to more cautious colleagues. This type of individual is extravert, optimistic, and enthusiastic who likes to be at the centre of attention and is a whirlwind of ideas.

- **The relater—the people person**
  This behavioural style demonstrates above-average responsiveness with comparatively low-level assertiveness. Such individuals are sympathetic and sensitive to the needs of others. Their altruistic qualities enable them to understand others more deeply. They employ the skills of empathy and understanding in interpersonal problem-solving situations. They are trusting and trustworthy, which enables them to bring out the best in their colleagues. Relaters are team players who like stability and who care greatly about relationships with others. They are amiable, often somewhat timid and slow to change, and generally resist direct confrontational involvement.

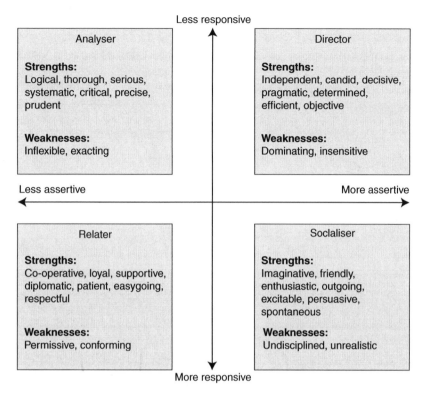

Figure 9.1 The strengths and weaknesses of each behavioural style adapted from Bolton and Bolton[1]

STRENGTHS AND WEAKNESSES OF EACH STYLE

The strengths and weaknesses of each behavioural style are summarised and shown in Figure 9.1. Usually an individual lacks the strengths of the style diagonally across the grid from his or her own style. An effective leadership team is composed of individuals from each of the quadrants in the table.

The behavioural style paradigm is an important reference point for evaluating team dynamics. The best and most productive interpersonal relationships and communications occur when two styles become complementary with each individual's strengths, thereby compensating for the weaknesses of the other.

STYLES WITHIN TEAMS AND ORGANISATIONS

The functional dynamics of a team are greatly affected by the styles of its members,[2] who in turn will impact directly on leadership. Leadership tasks require a combination of all four behavioural types in a manager.[3] Drucker also suggests that finding the strengths of all four types in one person is virtually impossible.

The most productive teams do, however, exhibit a balance of each of the behavioural styles amongst the team members. This gives rise to teams that will be more cohesive and able to work together for the benefit of the organisation. Moreover, an understanding of the behavioural style paradigm of all those involved assists with this interaction and facilitates a greater respect for the diversity within the group.

COMMUNICATION STYLES OF EACH CATEGORY

The preferred communication style of each category is shown in Table 9.1.

- **The analyser**—analysers prefer logical systematic conversations, not spontaneous impromptu reactions. They have a good attention spans and are good listeners. They are usually the conservative members of the organisation.

Table 9.1 Communication styles, limitations, and most preferred electronic communication style

Behavioural style	Preferred communication style	Personal limitations in communication	Preferred media
Analyser	Direct, formal, efficient economical. Meetings controlled by an agenda and minuted.	Inability to make use of flexible working. Unable to take advantage of informal networks, for example corridor conversations.	Formal e-mail. Formal telephone conversations.
Director	Adopt formal communication styles for formal and informal settings. Formal short meetings. Formal letters or memoranda.	Would not like others to alter or amend their contribution (for example, wikis). Not being in control. Would not like free communication. Would not allow digression or 'non-relevant contributions'	Formal e-mail. Telephone.
Relater	Informal. Opportunistic conversations (whether appropriate or not).	Not always able to adopt the most appropriate manner and behaviour in a specific forum, for example being flippant or humorous in formal meetings.	Informal e-mail. Telephone. Blogs. Wikis. Video/ teleconferences.
Socialiser	Informal. Opportunistic conversations (usually has social skills to assess appropriateness). Allows others to express themselves.	Keeping quiet. Allowing silences. Disciplined delivery of information.	E-mail. Wikis. Blogs. Telephone.

- **The director**—action-oriented directors have short attention spans, interrupt conversations, and avoid small talk. They have a pragmatic approach and are efficient and objective. Meetings are ideally short and to the point. The directors are the doers of the organisation.
- **The relater**—typically interested in others' lives, sensitive to moods and feelings, and would prefer to interact in social settings. Their offices will include comfortable chairs in which to sit and chat with tea- and coffee-making facilities. They are often considered the conscience of an organisation. They feel uncomfortable with behaviours that fail to take into consideration human elements.
- **The socialiser**—enthusiastic, imaginative, and idea people who may not have highly developed interpersonal skills. Their passion can sometimes make people feel uncomfortable in their presence and can be perceived as potentially volatile members.

For communication to be effective and productive, a combination of interpersonal relationships is desirable whereby the styles are complementary. The strengths of each can then be maximised and used to the benefit of the other party. When behavioural styles and communication abilities are understood, a synergistic relationship will develop.

This chapter has explored behavioural styles and identified the preferred communication media for each style.

And this shouldn't be a one-off; a note in your diary to check things three months or even a year later will pay dividends ('a way of involving others in your development …').

Should you run the questionnaire again? It might seem a good idea, but we would advise caution here. Questionnaires are subjective and interactive. In practice, this means that respondents compare you with their expectations of you. The first time around, this is new data. But a rerun of a questionnaire means that their expectations will have changed. It is not unusual for second-time-around scores to be *lower* rather than higher—not because the questioner is less effective, but because participants are sensitised and conditioned to expect more. So by all means, go around and ask but be wary about a simple rerun.

Finally, a familiar pattern in human nature, at least in British nature, is to focus on what we do badly and need to do less of. But another way of looking at feedback is to focus on what we do well and need to do more of. It may be that the feedback has highlighted certain strengths and a need to do them more. We should not forget the message implicit in the Belbin questionnaire, that each team role has strengths and weaknesses, but that the strengths and the weaknesses are closely bound up, and that the weaknesses are 'allowable'. So if you have had some positive feedback—particularly if it was unexpectedly positive—you might give yourself a moment of praise!

REFERENCES

1. Bolton R, Bolton D. *Social Style/Management Style*. New York. American Management Assoc.; 1984.
2. Hambrick D, Mason P. Upper echelons: the organization as a reflection of its tip-top managers. *Acad. Manage. Rev.* 1984; 9(2): 193–206.
3. Drucker P. *Management: tasks, responsibilities, and practices*. New York; Harper and Row; 1973.

CHAPTER 10

Adult learning and self-directed learners

Kay Mohanna, Elizabeth Cottrell, David Wall,
and Ruth Chambers

INTRODUCTION

Healthcare professionals are expected to be 'adult learners'—they will be independent and self-directed. Knowles coined the term 'androgogy' to refer to the art and science of teaching adults.[1]

Adult learning theory is built on five assumptions.[1]

1 Adults are independent and self-directing.
2 They have accumulated a great deal of experience, which is a rich resource for learning.
3 They value learning that integrates with the demands of their everyday life.
4 They are more interested in immediate, problem-centred approaches than in subject-centred ones.
5 They are more motivated to learn by internal drivers than by external ones.

Healthcare is too broad for all the content to be delivered by teachers. You must equip your learners with the skills to solve problems and continue learning throughout their careers:

> Education teaches us to solve problems, the nature of which may not be known to us at the time the education is taking place, and the solutions to which cannot be seen or even imagined by our teachers.[2]

Many people are frustrated by learners who do not behave as adults and expect to be 'spoon-fed'. Underlying this frustration is often a failure to recognise that the capacity to be self-directed is not an all-or-nothing function that develops overnight. Learners act at different levels or stages of self-direction depending on, for example, previous teaching, learning and assessment experiences, the subject matter, and the context of learning. Not all learners are ready to take responsibility for their own learning.

Effective teachers recognise this and realise that adult learning is *facilitated* by the teacher. Consider learning to be like a voyage in a boat. As the teacher, you do not stop being the rudder, but you avoid being the oars. Brookfield has debated the subject of adult learning at length, providing many examples.[3]

Grow's Staged Self-Directed Learning (SSDL) model builds on work by Hersey and is a helpful way to look at tensions that can arise if the learner's and teacher's levels are not matched.[4]

The SSDL model describes four developmental stages for students (S1–4):
1   dependent learner
2   interested learner
3   involved learner
4   self-directed learner.

and four styles of teaching (T1–4):
1   authority, coach
2   motivator, guide
3   facilitator
4   consultant, delegator.

For each learning stage, some ways of delivering teaching and activities are better suited than others (*see* Table 10.1).

Table 10.1 Stages of development of learning and teaching leading to self-directed learning

Stage or level of development of learner	Learner	Teacher	Examples of teaching activities
Stage 1	Dependent	Authority, coach	Coaching with immediate feedback Drill Informational lecture Overcoming deficiencies and resistance
Stage 2	Interested	Motivator, guide	Inspiring lecture plus guided discussion Goal-setting and learning strategies
Stage 3	Involved	Facilitator	Discussion facilitated by teacher who participates as equal Seminar Group projects
Stage 4	Self-directed	Consultant, delegator	Dissertation Individual work or self-directed study group

Table 10.2 Mismatch of levels of self-direction of learning with type of delivery of teaching

	T1: Authority Expert	T2: Motivator	T3: Facilitator	T4: Delegator
S4: Self-directed learner	Severe mismatch Students resent authoritarian teacher	*Mismatch*	Near match	Match
S3: Involved learner	*Mismatch*	Near match	Match	Near match
S2: Interested learner	Near match	Match	Near match	*Mismatch*
S1: Dependent learner	Match	Near match	*Mismatch*	Severe mismatch Learners resent freedom they are not ready for

Tensions can arise if the learner's stage and delivery of teaching are mismatched—for example, when dependent learners are placed with non-directive teachers and when self-directed learners work with highly directive teachers (*see* Table 10.2).

T1/S4 MISMATCH

When self-directed students (S4) are paired with an authoritarian teacher (T1), problems may arise, although some S4 learners develop the ability to function well and retain overall control of their learning, even under directive teachers. However, other S4 learners will resent the authoritarian teacher and rebel against the barrage of low-level demands. This mismatch may cause the learner to rebel or to retreat into boredom. Furthermore, the T1 teacher will probably not interpret such rebellion as the result of a mismatch. Instead, that teacher is likely to see the learner as surly, uncooperative, and unprepared to concentrate on learning basic facts. Extreme overcontrol by any leader results in stress and conflict, and in the follower engaging in behaviour designed to get the leader out—or to escape from under the leader.

T1/S3–S4 MISMATCH

Learners who are capable of more individual involvement in learning are relegated to passive roles in authoritarian classrooms.

Adults who return to education may find themselves in this position. Their life experiences and learning skills generally enable them to learn at the S3 or S4 level, but they may be placed with teachers accustomed to using Stage 1 and 2 methods on adolescents.

Furthermore, after many years of responsibility, adults may experience difficulty learning from T1 teachers. Adults may be accustomed to having authority and are unused to blindly doing what they are told without understanding why and consenting to the task.

Adults returning for postgraduate study, in particular, may run aground on courses like statistics, which are often taught by briskly directive teachers using the Stage 1 mode. The more appropriate Stage 3 mode is not always used with older learners when teachers lack experience in this type of teaching.

T4/S1 MISMATCH

When dependent learners (S1) are paired with a T3 or T4 teacher, they may be delegated responsibility for learning that they are not equipped to handle.

Such learners may be unable to make use of the 'freedom to learn' because they lack the following necessary skills for self-directed learning:

- goal setting
- self-evaluation
- project management
- critical thinking
- group participation
- learning strategies
- information resources
- self-esteem.

Learners may resent the teacher for forcing upon them a freedom for which they are not ready. These dependent learners expect close supervision, immediate feedback, frequent interaction, constant motivation, and the reassuring presence of an authority figure telling them what to do. Such learners are unlikely to respond well to the delegating style of teaching, a hands-off delegator, or a critical theorist who demands that they confront their own learning roles.

Grow describes the results of this mismatch as a kind of 'havoc' that occurs when the followers do not receive the guidance that they need, and:

> 'Lacking the ability to perform the task, [they] tend to feel that the leader has little interest in their work and does not care about them personally. [This form of teacher leadership makes] it difficult for these followers to increase their ability, and reinforces their lack of confidence. If the leader waits too long but then provides high amounts of structure, the followers tend to see this action as a punitive rather than a helping relationship'.[4]

The learner's stage of self-direction is often a result of the teaching that they have previously experienced. Consider the following:

'I am the product of a system built around assignments, deadlines, and conventional examinations. Therefore, with this course graded by the flexible method and four other courses graded by the more conventional methods, I tend to give less attention to this course than it merits, due to a lack of well-defined requirements'.

This learner has made a strategic decision about study. Other learners in this position may experience shock and resentment when faced with the necessity of making unguided, responsible choices.

THE FALSE STAGE 4 LEARNER

Some students appear to be Stage 4 self-directed learners, but turn out to be highly dependent students in a state of defiance. The one who shouts loudest, 'No! I'll do it *my* way!' is likely to be a 'false independent' learner who may resist mastering the necessary details of the subject and 'wing it' at an abstract level.

False independent learners need help to raise their knowledge and skills to the level of their self-belief. They may need to master how to learn productively from others, and may benefit from a strong-willed teacher who challenges them to become autonomous and effective.

DEPENDENT, RESISTANT LEARNERS AS A PRODUCT OF THE EDUCATIONAL SYSTEM

The way in which undergraduates are often taught can produce learners who resist direction. A group of highly resistant learners can coerce teachers into an authoritarian mode, and then frustrate them, at the same time being dependent on teachers and resentful of being taught.

The resistant form of Stage 1 is probably not a natural condition. It results from years of dependency training. Most children are naturally Stage 3 or 4 learners when undirected. Even when taught in a directive manner, they are generally available, interested, and excitable, and have a spontaneous creative energy that they are willing to direct into satisfying projects under the guidance of a capable teacher.

Resistant-dependent learning may be a product of culture and upbringing, as well as of the education system. Sources of resistance in adult learners may include threats to cultural identity that might have been generated by the (hopefully now changing) pressures of hierarchical medicine. You need to understand dependency in context—certain forms of help may make the problem worse.

USING THE SSDL MODEL IN PRACTICE

As outlined above, the SSDL model describes four styles of teaching (T1-4).

Box 10.1 Knowles' guidelines on teaching self-directed adults

Knowles defined seven fundamentals that have stood the test of time as guidelines to encourage adult learners.[1]

1 Establish an effective learning climate in which learners feel safe and comfortable expressing themselves.
2 Involve learners in mutual planning of relevant methods and curricular content.
3 Trigger internal motivation by involving learners in diagnosing their own needs.
4 Give learners more control by encouraging them to formulate their own learning objectives.
5 Encourage learners to identify resources and devise strategies for using resources to achieve their objectives.
6 Support learners in carrying out their learning plans.
7 Develop learners' skills of critical reflection by involving them in evaluating their own learning.

Following these guidelines might encourage learners to move up through the stages.

BROOKFIELD'S PRINCIPLES OF ADULT LEARNING

There are six principles of adult learning that you should build into your teaching.[3]

1 **Participation is voluntary**—the decision to learn is that of the learner.
2 **There should be mutual respect**—shown by teachers and learners for each other, and by learners for other learners.
3 **Collaboration is important**—between learners and teachers, and among learners.
4 **Action and reflection**—learning is a continuous process of investigation, exploration, action, reflection, and further action.
5 **Critical reflection**—this brings awareness that alternatives can be presented as challenges to the learner to gather evidence, ask questions, and develop a critically aware frame of mind.
6 **Self-directed adult individuals need to be nurtured.**

HOW TO PUT THE PRINCIPLES OF ADULT LEARNING INTO PRACTICE

What can busy healthcare professionals do to help themselves and their learners to develop into self-directed, independent adult learners? Brookfield gives 10 tips on doing this (*see* Box 10.2).

Box 10.2 How to create an adult learner

1 Progressively reduce the learner's dependence on the teachers.
2 Help the learner to understand the use of learning resources, including the experiences of fellow learners.
3 Help the learner to use reflective practice to define their learning needs.
4 Help the learner to define their learning objectives, plan their programmes, and assess their own progress.
5 Organise what is to be learned in terms of personal understanding, goals, and concerns at the learner's level of understanding.
6 Encourage the learner to take decisions and to expand their learning experiences and range of opportunities for learning.
7 Encourage the use of criteria for judging all aspects of learning, not just those that are easy to measure.
8 Facilitate problem posing and problem solving in relation to personal and group needs issues.
9 Reinforce progressive mastery of skills through constructive feedback and mutual support.
10 Emphasise experiential learning (learning by doing, learning on the job) and the use of learning contracts.

WORK-BASED LEARNING

Work-based learning aligns with the principles of adult learning and represents the most accessible opportunities for self-directed learning during clinical work. Clinical experiences offer a vast range of learning opportunities. Encourage self-directed work-based learning by promoting and enhancing the quality of:

• reflection
• management of complaints
• significant events and critical incidents
• audit
• handover.

Reflection

All healthcare practitioners and teachers should regularly reflect on their practice. Formal evidence of reflection is required for clinical and academic professional portfolios, and these skills are often sought in job-recruitment processes. Learners sometimes struggle to see the worth of reflection and, anecdotally, this can be a problem among undergraduates. You must undertake regular reflection on your own work, be able to assist learners with reflection, and highlight the benefits of doing so.

Why reflect?

The important benefits of reflection are as follows:
- keeping abreast of changes to the healthcare system, patient expectations, and/ or medical knowledge
- helping to understand why things went well or why they didn't—this can help both clinical practice and self-esteem, particularly if things have gone wrong
- helping you to make sense of a difficult situation, to prevent a knee-jerk reaction and unfair attribution of causation
- improving practice for the next time by taking a more informed and thought-out approach
- identifying learning needs to direct progress with personal-development plans.

Although documented evidence of formal reflective practice is usually required, not all reflection needs to be written down. Take learners through the process of reflection through discussion (e.g. of a specific case or after role play).

Models of reflection

Reflection is about dissecting a situation and understanding the whys and the hows, rather than just stating what happened. A number of models outline stages of reflection:
- Gibbs' model of reflection (1988)[6]
- Johns' model of reflection (1994)[7]
- Atkins and Murphy's model of reflection (1994)[8]
- Holm and Stephenson's model of reflection (1994).[9]

Figure 10.1 summarises the key points from each to provide a cycle of prompts and processes that should be considered for effective reflection. However, not all of them may be applicable in every case.

Study as cases or questions arise

Reflection in action can be encouraged by teachers until it becomes self-directed. For example, in the clinical environment, a learner may detect a condition that they have little experience of managing. Rather than stepping in and taking over, you can establish what the learner already knows and encourage them to address any knowledge gaps. Learners could try a management approach or research missing knowledge in the clinical setting, for example, by consulting evidence-based guidelines. This helps the learner to reach a conclusion through careful reasoning. The learner can direct their subsequent personal study to read up about their case and any remaining knowledge deficits. Maintaining a notebook to record questions, uncertainties, or knowledge gaps may ensure that personal study can be directed appropriately.[10]

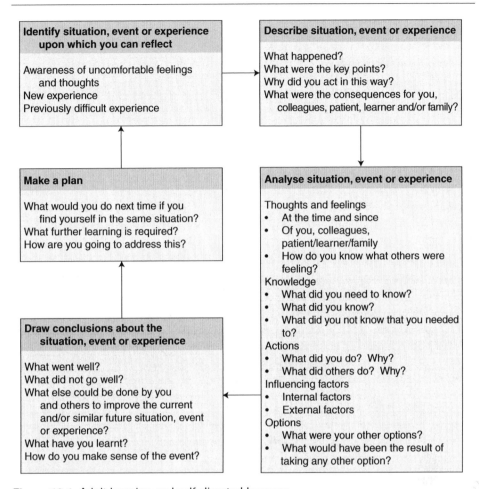

Figure 10.1 Adult learning and self-directed learners

Following up cases that have been seen

To promote *reflection on action* and to prevent worthwhile reflective cases or situations being missed, learners should be encouraged to follow up cases that they have seen. Often the cases in which unforeseen circumstances arose are those from which the most can be learned. This may not necessarily mean that a mistake occurred, but rather that a patient's condition was not what it first appeared to be, or problems within healthcare system delivery prevented the originally planned management. Such cases may not be routinely brought to the attention of the learner if no mistakes were made or the patient has not been harmed. However, for the learner, there may be a wealth of learning opportunities to address. The self-directed learner will take note of the patients they see and find out what subsequently happens during the care episode. Any cases in which unforeseen circumstances arose could be used for a significant event analysis

Complaints

You may feel defensive, disheartened, and/or defeated upon receiving a complaint. However, complaints can be a useful stimulus for reflection and professional development. All professionals have to answer complaints that arise against them. As a junior, this may consist of providing a statement to senior staff, who may handle the situation from then on, or a formal response may be required. The skills learned through developing your reflective practice will assist with the production of such documents and also with the explanations that are provided to patients. Maintaining a complaints record aids detection of any patterns of problems.[11] You should help learners to consolidate what they have learned from a complaint by considering the following:[12]

- description of the event
- concerns expressed by the complainant
- assessment of the complaint
- actions resulting from the assessment
- outcome, including the response to the complainant
- reflection on the experience and a description of the learner's own involvement.

Significant events and critical incidents

Significant event analyses and critical incident reporting are increasingly becoming ingrained in the normal working practice of every healthcare professional, and are recognised conduits for identifying problems in services, initiating change to improve the quality of practice and patient safety, and influencing professional development through reflective learning.[12, 13] Significant events are cases in which an adverse, unforeseen, or undesired—clinical, administrative, or teaching—event has occurred. Often they involve situations in which harm or potential harm has resulted, but they do not necessarily do so. Therefore, significant event analysis, which is a qualitative method of clinical audit that is undertaken on an individual case basis, has become a core component of work for many healthcare professionals, and is commonly required for appraisal, revalidation, and professional accreditation.[14] Although the term 'critical incident' may be synonymous with 'significant event', it can also describe situations that the professional has identified as being important in their professional development. Thus, the event may not have posed a threat to patient safety, but may have been challenging or particularly rich in learning points. The latter situation should be addressed in the same manner as reflection (*see* Figure 10.1).

The following steps are involved in significant event analysis:[14, 15]

1 identify the significant event for analysis
2 collect and collate data, including both factual information and gathering the thoughts, opinions, and impressions of those involved

3   organise a meeting of relevant team members to discuss and analyse the signifi-
    cant event
4   agree and implement changes and organise follow-up
5   keep a written record
6   obtain peer review of the process and outcomes.

Formal reporting and analysis of significant events and critical incidents, like the
management of complaints, are tasks that require good reflective skills and are useful catalysts for learning. The same prompts can be used during steps 2–4 of a significant event analysis as are provided for reflection (*see* Figure 10.1). However, the
involved team must participate in discussions and analysis of the event. Evidence
that changes have occurred and the results of these changes are also usually
required when reporting significant events, particularly for appraisal or revalidation
purposes.[12]

Audit

Audit is the process whereby actual practice—organisational, clinical, or educational—is compared with predefined standards and/or expectations of practice.
In contrast to the individual case nature of significant event analysis, audits examine data of multiple cases, procedures, or actions in order to obtain an overview
of service provision. Data regarding your personal or service's practice are gathered and compared with the expected, predefined standards, and any deficits are
identified. Formal reflection can help to explain areas that require attention and/
or improvement to better meet the standards, and a plan should be made to
initiate change. Once the change has been initiated, the whole process should
be repeated to establish signs of improvement in adherence to expected practice.
Thus a cycle is created that should be worked around repeatedly. You should assist
your learners to undertake audit, and you should audit your own clinical and/or
educational practice.

Handovers

Handovers are an excellent opportunity for work-based learning. They affect clinical
care, and due to shortened working hours, they have become increasingly frequent.
Handovers can be the weak link of the patient care chain. Failure to hand over
adequately can result in clinical errors, wasted time and/or money, poor patient
care, patient dissatisfaction, and potentially patient death. Help learners to identify areas for development through robust and informative handover processes.
Formal handovers involving seniors at each shift change provide an ideal platform
for ensuring appropriate and adequate handover by junior staff and for questioning
and exploring patient management.

Box 10.3 Tips from experienced teachers

Consistent reflection is the single most important skill to impart to a learner. It will lead to a change in attitudes as well as updated knowledge and new technical skills, and will enable them to maintain a consistently good performance throughout their health professional career.

REFERENCES

1. Knowles MS. *Androgogy in Action: applying modern principles of adult learning.* San Francisco, CA: Jossey-Bass; 1984.
2. Marinker M. Assessment of postgraduate medical education—future directions. In: Lawrence M and Pritchard P, editors. *General Practice Education: UK and Nordic perspectives.* London: Springer Verlag; 1992.
3. Brookfield SD. *Understanding and Facilitating Adult Learning.* Milton Keynes: Open University Press; 1986.
4. Grow GO. Teaching learners to be self-directed. *Adult Educ Quart.* 1996; **41**(3): 125–49.
5. Schon DA. *Educating the Reflective Practitioner: toward a new design for teaching and learning in the professions.* San Francisco, CA: Jossey-Bass; 1987.
6. Gibbs G. *Learning by Doing: a guide to teaching and learning methods.* Oxford: Further Education Unit, Oxford Polytechnic; 1988.
7. Johns C. Framing learning through reflection within Carper's fundamental ways of knowing in nursing. *J Adv Nurs.* 1995; **22**: 226–34.
8. Atkins S, Murphy K. Reflective practice. *Nurs Stand.* 1994; **8**: 49–56.
9. Palmer A, Burns S, Bulman C, editors. *Reflective Practice in Nursing: the growth of the professional practitioner.* Oxford: Blackwell Scientific Publications; 1994.
10. Johnson C, Bird J. How to Teach Reflective Practice Cardiff. Cardiff University School of Post Graduate Medical and Dental Education. www.cardiff.ac.uk/pgmde/resources/howtoreflective.pdf
11. Royal College of General Practitioners. *RCGP Guide to the Revalidation of General Practitioners Version 3.* London: Royal College of General Practitioners. 2010.
12. Branch WT. List of Critical Incident Reports in Medical Education. *J Gen Intern Med.* 2005; **20**: 1063–67.
13. Bowie P, Mc Kay A, Dalgetty E. et al. A Qualitative Study of Why General Practitioners May Participate in Significant Event Analysis and Educational Peer Assessment. *Qual Saf Health Care.* 2005; **14**: 185–89.
14. NHS Education for Scotland. Significant Event Analysis. www.Nes.scot.nhs.uk/pharmacy/CPD/SEA.
15. Pringle M, Bradley CP, Carmichael CM, et al. Significant Event Auditing, A Study of the Feasibility and Potential of Case- Based Auditing in Primary Medical Care. *Occas Pap R Col Gen Pract.* 1995; **79**(i–viii): 1–71.

CHAPTER 11

Developing your teaching style and techniques

Kay Mohanna, Elizabeth Cottrell, David Wall, and Ruth Chambers

INTRODUCTION

This chapter will help you to understand your natural teaching style and consider how to adapt it to various learners' needs to help them progress from being dependent to self-directed learners. Just as the learner has a favoured learning style, you will have a preferred teaching style. Your teaching style has a powerful effect on the dynamics of their learning experience. Thus, you should adapt it or adopt more appropriate styles according to the purpose of your teaching.

An effective teacher does not just impart knowledge and skills, but does so in a way that engages learners and leaves them with a deeper understanding and ability to interpret that freshly gained knowledge, or to apply those new skills. The effective teacher empowers a student to want to learn more, to actually do so, and to put their learning into practice.

BE AWARE OF YOUR OWN TEACHING STYLE(S)

Your appearance, voice, and what you say are vitally important in addition to your teaching style. Your gestures and body language should not be distracting, and should complement your voice and the messages of your teaching.

You will have developed your teaching style as a result of what comes naturally to you, the training and feedback that you have received, and your experience. There may have been some particular role models who have influenced your style, as you have unconsciously emulated teachers whom you have found inspiring, or deliberately avoided being like those with an off-putting style. You might have a quiet, introverted personality and tend toward the *all-around flexible and adaptable* teaching style, or you may be an extravert and enjoy the *big conference* teaching style. Your healthcare discipline may also influence your teaching style. Doctors often adopt a dominating style and expect to be in charge, whereas nurses and allied health professionals may be more learner-centred.

You will become more aware of the nature of the style that you are using and how effective it is from continuing reflection, feedback, and evaluation of your teaching over the years. However, good performance requires a supportive teaching environment, sufficient time to deliver the required scope and level of learning, a reasonable teacher/learner ratio, and a good match between learners' needs and your expertise/knowledge. Non-work-related worries, such as health or financial concerns, working in unfamiliar settings, or being generally harassed, may affect your performance and awareness of your teaching style. These factors may affect your concentration, restrict your intuitive powers, and limit your reflective insights.

You may not feel comfortable using all teaching styles. However, your ability to vary your teaching style according to learners' needs and level(s) and the purpose of the learning activity will depend on your insight. Exploit those styles that you are good at, and practise the other styles for delivering learning when there is minimal pressure and you can obtain constructive feedback.

INVESTIGATE YOUR TEACHING STYLE

One way of considering the varied range of teaching styles is the Staffordshire Evaluation of Teaching Styles (SETS) approach.[1] The underpinning research determined six main styles.

1 **The all-round flexible and adaptable teacher** can use many different skills, can teach both peers and juniors, and is very aware of the whole environment both of teaching and of the learners.
2 **The student-centred, sensitive teacher** is very learner-centred, teaches in small groups, with emotions to the fore, using role-play and drama, and is not comfortable doing straight presentations.
3 **The official formal curriculum teacher** is very well prepared, accredited, is very aware of and adheres to the formal curriculum, and follows external targets.
4 **The straight-facts, no-nonsense teacher** likes to teach the clear facts, with straight talking, concentrating on specific skills, and much prefers not to be involved with multi-professional teaching and learning.
5 **The big conference teacher** most enjoys standing up in front of a large audience, and does not like sitting in groups or one-to-one teaching.
6 **The one-off teacher** likes to deliver small self-contained topics, on a one-to-one basis, with no props to help and no follow-up.

Try working out your preferred teaching style(s) by completing the four steps of the next exercise.

- **Step 1.** Fill in the questionnaire.
- **Step 2.** Score your answers.
- **Step 3.** Rate each of the six teaching styles.
- **Step 4.** Plot your ratings to compare and contrast your preferences for each of the six teaching styles.

STEP 1: WORK OUT YOUR PREFERRED TEACHING STYLE(S) BY ANSWERING THE FOLLOWING QUESTIONS

Rate the extent to which you agree with each of the statements below from 1 (do not agree at all) to 5 (very strongly agree).

	Do not agree at all				Very strongly agree
Q1. I vary my approach depending on my audience	1	2	3	4	5
Q2. I am less comfortable giving straight presentations than teaching through games and exercises	1	2	3	4	5
Q3. I prefer to teach through games to relay learning	1	2	3	4	5
Q4. I like having external targets to determine the course of learning	1	2	3	4	5
Q5. I prefer teaching sessions that are self-contained with no follow-up	1	2	3	4	5
Q6. Props often detract from a talk	1	2	3	4	5
Q7. I am comfortable addressing large audiences	1	2	3	4	5
Q8. Preparation for my teaching focuses on me and my role	1	2	3	4	5
Q9. I am usually standing up when I teach	1	2	3	4	5
Q10. The best teaching sessions convey straight facts in a clear way	1	2	3	4	5
Q11. I avoid being distracted from running sessions the way I plan to run them	1	2	3	4	5
Q12. I am happy teaching general skills	1	2	3	4	5
Q13. I put no value on being formally employed as a teacher	1	2	3	4	5
Q14. I dislike one-to-one (tutor) teaching	1	2	3	4	5
Q15. I am consistent in delivery of a topic, whatever the audience	1	2	3	4	5

(Continued)

	Do not agree at all				Very strongly agree
Q16. I like to give students the opportunity to explore how to learn	**1**	**2**	**3**	**4**	**5**
Q17. I have developed my own style as a teacher	**1**	**2**	**3**	**4**	**5**
Q18. I prefer one-to-one (tutor) teaching	**1**	**2**	**3**	**4**	**5**
Q19. Eliciting emotions through role play or drama is a valuable aspect of teaching	**1**	**2**	**3**	**4**	**5**
Q20. I am comfortable using humour in my teaching	**1**	**2**	**3**	**4**	**5**
Q21. I am rarely sitting down when teaching students	**1**	**2**	**3**	**4**	**5**
Q22. It is important to me that my teaching is accredited by an official body	**1**	**2**	**3**	**4**	**5**
Q23. I am uncomfortable when I have multi-professional groups of learners to teach	**1**	**2**	**3**	**4**	**5**
Q24. I am at my best when organising my teaching to fit an external curriculum or organisational structure	**1**	**2**	**3**	**4**	**5**

STEP 2: COMPLETE YOUR SCORING GRID

Write your score for each of the questions in the correct boxes, then add up the columns to obtain your score for each of the six teaching styles (out of a maximum of 20 marks).

Question	Style 1	Style 2	Style 3	Style 4	Style 5	Style 6
Q1	Q1 =					
Q2		Q2 =				
Q3		Q3 =				
Q4			Q4 =			
Q5						Q5 =
Q6						Q6 =
Q7					Q7 =	
Q8/		Q8 =				
Q9					Q9 =	
Q10				Q10 =		
Q11				Q11 =		
Q12	Q12 =					
Q13						Q13 =

(*Continued*)

Question	Style 1	Style 2	Style 3	Style 4	Style 5	Style 6
Q14					Q14 =	
Q15				Q15 =		
Q16		Q16 =				
Q17	Q17 =					
Q18						Q18 =
Q19		Q19 =				
Q20	Q20 =					
Q21					Q21 =	
Q22			Q22 =			
Q23				Q23 =		
Q24			Q24 =			
Totals						

STEP 3: RATE EACH TEACHING STYLE

Fill in your scores, obtained from the chart totals in Step 2, in the six boxes against each of the teaching styles listed below.

		Your scores
Style 1	The all-around flexible and adaptable teacher	
Style 2	The student-centred, sensitive teacher	
Style 3	The official formal curriculum teacher	
Style 4	The straight-facts, no-nonsense teacher	
Style 5	The big conference teacher	
Style 6	The one-off teacher	

Now you have the six scores out of 20 for your self-evaluation of your preferred teaching styles.

STEP 4: PLOT YOUR PREFERRED TEACHING STYLE(S) ON THE SETS HEXAGON

Plot the marks from the rating sheet in Step 3 with a cross along each of the six axes to represent your score for each of the six teaching styles. Join up the crosses to produce a shape that represents your own combination of styles.

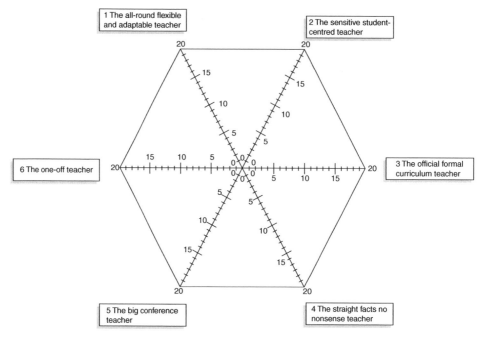

Figure 11.1 Your preferred teaching style(s)

TAILORING YOUR TEACHING STYLE(S) TO STUDENTS' LEARNING STYLE(S)

Consider whether your preferred teaching style suits the learning style(s) and needs of your learners for particular teaching episodes. If it does not, you should switch or adapt your teaching style to engage with your learners better and, hopefully, to improve their understanding, knowledge, and skills. The main approaches to tailoring your teaching style to learners' needs are summarised below.

Matching

This will encourage learners to be interested and involved. Introverts prefer well-structured situations, so a *straight facts, no-nonsense* teaching style might suit this type of learner. Extraverts prefer less structured situations, so the *all-around flexible and adaptable* teaching style should be suitable for these learners.

Allowing choice

The *all-round flexible and adaptable* teaching style should suit learners from a range of backgrounds and with various levels of knowledge and skills, as you vary your style and content to match their needs and preferences. You should guide them in an engaging way using your *sensitive, student-centred* style.

Table 11.1 Teaching delivery matched against the six SETS teaching styles

Teaching delivery	SETS teaching styles					
	All-round flexible	Student-centred	Official curriculum	Straight facts	Big conference	One-off
Authority	✓		✓	✓	✓	
Motivator	✓	✓	maybe		maybe	maybe
Facilitator	✓	✓				✓
Delegator	✓	✓				✓

Providing several different methods of learning on the same course

If this approach is used, all of the learners should find something that suits them during the course, whether they are dependent, interested, involved, or self-directed learners. The *all-around flexible and adaptable* teaching style fits well, as it motivates and guides interested and involved learners. The *sensitive, student-centred* teacher will craft their teaching to the various learning styles of a group of learners and the specific needs of individual learners, handling dependent learners as well as firing up self-directed learners. The *official curriculum* teaching style is more authoritarian and will be useful for covering the formal content of a course required for accreditation. The *big conference* teaching style could be useful for providing variety to all kinds of learners, and a *one-off* teaching style might make the most of experts brought in as external speakers. The *straight facts, no-nonsense* style could help during revision sessions for dependent learners or for students who are falling behind in their course work.

Independent study for self-directed learners

The *all-around flexible and adaptable* teacher will facilitate and encourage the freedom to study as independent learning, especially with more mature learners.

MATCHING YOUR TEACHING STYLE TO LEARNERS' NEEDS AND PREFERENCES

Another way of thinking about different teaching styles relates to your teaching *personality*. We shall return to Grow's stages of self-directed learning (SSDL) model with four types of delivery of teaching:[2, 3]

1   T1: authority; coach
2   T2: motivator; guide
3   T3: facilitator
4   T4: consultant; delegator.

You need various types of teaching delivery described in the SSDL model for the six teaching styles of the SETS model. Different ways of delivering teaching (authoritarian, motivational, facilitatory, and delegator) can be applied to the six different SETS teaching styles and situations (*see* Table 11.1).

The SSDL model suggests why 'good teaching' is widely misunderstood. Often people think that there is only one way to teach well—and usually it is their way!

Awards generally go to teachers who are outstanding in one of the first two stages, either the one who provides copious structured information and instruction (sometimes called 'bucket filling', where the learner is seen as a vessel ready to be filled with information from the teacher) or the one who leads and motivates learners. Awards less often go to teachers who encourage learners to develop independently, or those who engage the most advanced learners with deep, open-ended problems.

'Good teaching' for one learner may not be 'good teaching' for another, or even for the same learner at a different stage of development. Good teaching does two things. It matches the learner's stage of self-direction and it empowers the learner to progress toward greater self-direction. Good teaching is situational, yet it promotes the long-term development of the learner.

MISMATCH BETWEEN TEACHING STYLE AND STAGE OF LEARNING

Even if adult teachers recognise that adult learners are not all necessarily self-directed learners, it is widely assumed that adults will become self-directed after a few sessions of explaining the concept.

However, not all adults become self-directed just because they have been told to do so. Adult learners can be at any of the four learning stages, but the literature on adult education is dominated by advocates of what the SSDL model would call a Stage 3 method—a facilitative approach, emphasising group activity. However, teachers may sometimes need to approach certain learners in a directive, authoritarian style, and then gradually equip those learners with the skills, self-concept, and motivation necessary to pursue learning in a more self-directed manner.

Advocates of a classroom in which learner and teacher receive equal respect acknowledge the paradoxical need to be directive, as Grow states:

'On the one hand, I cannot manipulate. On the other hand, I cannot leave the students by themselves. The opposite of these two possibilities is being radically democratic. That means accepting the directive nature of education. There is a directiveness in education which never allows it to be neutral. My role is not to be silent'.[2]

Every stage involves balancing the teacher's power with the learner's emerging self-direction.

The temptations of each teaching style

The temptation for the Stage 1 teacher is to be authoritarian in a punitive, controlling way that stifles initiative and creates resistance and dependency.

The temptation for the Stage 2 teacher is to remain on centre stage, inspiring all who will listen but leaving them with no more learning skills or self-motivation than when they started.

The Stage 3 teacher can disappear into the group and demoralise learners by 'accepting and valuing almost anything from anybody'.

The Stage 4 teacher can withdraw too much from the learning experience, lose touch, fail to monitor progress, and let learners hang themselves with rope they are not yet accustomed to handling.

In each instance, the teacher may falter in the immensely difficult juggling act of becoming 'vitally, vigorously, creatively, energetically, and inspiringly unnecessary'.

Recursive teaching

The SSDL model describes a progression of stages, but the progress of a learner or class will rarely be linear, and most classes will contain learners at different stages of self-direction. A more realistic version of the model would be non-linear and iterative.

Consider a course designed according to the Stage 3 model. The teacher serves as group facilitator, with the job of empowering learners to take greater charge of their learning and making certain that they master advanced levels of the subject matter. Most of the work takes place in the Stage 3 arena, where the teacher attempts to phase out external leadership and empower more self-direction.

However, there will be times when other learning modes are necessary. When the group—or some of its members—is deficient in basic skills, they may require drill and practice, a Stage 1 approach. Even advanced learners sometimes choose T1 teachers who push them to achieve goals that they cannot achieve under their own motivation. Sometimes the T3 teacher may determine that coaching or confrontation is necessary to reach a learner. The class may loop back to the Stage 1 mode for a while before returning to Stage 3.

Continued motivation and encouragement may sometimes be supplied by members of the class, but it may require the teacher to shift to the Stage 2 mode and provide it.

At times, the teacher's knowledge matters more than anything else; lecturing may be the best possible response at that point. During the lecture, the class loops back to the Stage 1 or Stage 2 mode, and then returns to the group interaction and subtle facilitation of the Stage 3 mode.

When individuals or subgroups become ready to exert self-direction and leadership, these learners can go into the S4 mode, independently carry out a project and then come back to the group and teach the results. With the Stage 3 facilitated mode of teaching as a base, the class can loop out to the other three stages when appropriate.

Box 11.1 Tips from experienced teachers
- Don't become lazy. Continue to adapt your teaching style for your learners, and put their needs first.
- Specify the requirements for an assignment in a supportive way so that dependent learners can more easily progress to being self-directed as they plan and apply their newly acquired knowledge and skills.
- Stay humble. Welcome all feedback from learners (especially that which you could not have predicted), and continue to reflect on how you might improve your future delivery of teaching to different groups of learners.
- Listen, listen, listen … to your learners.

A class that is focused on any stage of learning from S1 to S4 can draw support from the earlier stages and lean toward the later stages. Many courses centre around a series of Stage 1/Stage 2 lectures, but have a weekly discussion group that is more in the Stage 3 mode. 'Looping' may be a more effective way to use the SSDL concept than trying to follow a sequence of linear stages.

REFERENCES

1. Mohanna K, Chambers R, Wall D. *Your Teaching Style; a practical guide to understanding, developing and improving.* Oxford: Radcliffe Publishing; 2008.
2. Grow GP. Teaching learners to be self-directed. *Adult Educ Quarterly.* 1996; **41**: 125–49.
3. www.longleaf.net/ggrow.

FURTHER READING

- Bennett SN. *Teaching Styles and Pupil Progress.* London: Open Books; 1976.
- Butler KA. *Learning and Teaching Style: in theory and practice.* Columbia, CT: The Learner's Dimension; 1984.
- Entwistle NJ. *Styles of Learning and Teaching.* London: David Fulton Publishers; 1988.
- Kaufman DM, Mann KV, Jennett PA. *Teaching and Learning in Medical Education: how theory can inform practice.* Edinburgh: Association for the Study of Medical Education; 2000.

CHAPTER 12

Models, techniques, and approaches for change management

Robert Jones and Fiona Jenkins

Everything flows and nothing stays
You can't step twice into the same river[1]

INTRODUCTION

Change is an every day occurrence for all healthcare staff whether managers, clinicians, or members of support teams. The way in which change is embraced and managed impacts on the care provided for patients as well as the success of organisations, services, and personal job satisfaction. As managers and leaders of healthcare services, it is imperative that we have an understanding of the theoretical concepts of change management and the practical skills to lead and manage change. Our aim in this chapter is to provide an overview and insight into this important sphere of management, to introduce and focus on our 'Framework for the Management of Change', and to set out a case study that is an example of successful change management projects based on the 'Framework' and from our own experience as managers and leaders in the AHPs and wider healthcare. The chapter also relates closely to Chapter 14 in this volume, which is focused on the development of care pathways incorporating many elements of change management and leadership.

Throughout the last hundred years, academics and practitioners have developed a very extensive body of literature on the theory and practice of change management, including the development of a wide range of concepts, models, tools, and techniques—there are many schools of thought with an ever-increasing literature supporting the evidence base. For this reason, it has not been possible here to set out a detailed analysis of this vast and complex field of theory and practice, but to provide a selective review and positive guidance.

CHANGE

Everyone finds change difficult; according to Samuel Johnson,[2] 'Change is not made without inconvenience, even from worse to better,' and it is clear from the literature on the management and leadership of change that there is no 'right' 'best' or only one way of doing it. Bernard Burnes[3] recognises that what almost everyone would like is a clear and practical change theory that explains what changes organisations need to make and how they should make them. Unfortunately, what is available is a wide range of confusing and contradictory theories, approaches, and recipes. Many of these are well thought out and grounded in both theory and practice; others, unfortunately, seem disconnected from either theory or reality. Also, though change theory requires an interdisciplinary perspective, each of the major approaches tends to view organisations from the disciplinary angles of their originators—whether it be psychology, sociology, economics, or whatever—which can result in an incomplete and biased picture. So, regardless of what their proponents may claim, we do not possess at present an approach to change that is theoretically holistic, universally applicable, and which can be practically applied.

Change management is not a distinct discipline with rigid and clearly defined boundaries, but rather the theory and practice draws on a wide range of social science disciplines and traditions. Something that is certain is that all of us—whoever we are and whatever we do—are involved in, subject to, and bringers about of change in the working environment whatever our roles, grades, or professions.

Change is one of the few constants of recorded history.[1, 2]

Often society's 'winners', both historical and contemporary, can be characterised by their common ability to effectively manage and exploit change situations. Management and change are synonymous, and it is impossible to undertake a journey—for in many respects, that is what change is—without first addressing the purpose of the trip, the route you wish to travel, and with whom.[4]

There are many elements that make up the 'jigsaw of reform' with very significant implications for AHPs and all other NHS managers and staff, including, for example:
- developing service commissioning and accountability
- performance management
- reducing risk
- maintaining financial control
- developing service providers—including the 'third sector'
- developing the workforce
- the changing legal and regulatory framework.

It is clear from these examples that the pace and intensity of change will continue unabated and will continue to affect all those working in healthcare; it is therefore essential that managers and staff from all backgrounds develop strategies for proactively managing and leading, handling, and participating in change processes.

Change management can be approached from a variety of different angles and applied to numerous organisational processes. To be effective, it needs to be multidisciplinary, touching all aspects of the organisation. An essential element in implementing new procedures, technologies, ways of working, and overcoming resistance to change is through effective involvement of all. A complex interplay of emotions and cognitive processes bear on attitudes to change; people therefore react to change differently. On the positive side, change may be seen as opportunity, renewal, rejuvenation, progress, innovation, or growth whilst on the other hand—and equally legitimately—it might be seen as upheaval, instability, threat, disorientation, and unpredictability. Whether change is perceived as frightening, demoralising, or the source of anxiety and stress or is approached with excitement, enthusiasm, confidence, or somewhere between these is dependent on many factors, including the psychological make up of individuals, the actions of managers and leaders, the behaviour and ethos of the organisation or service, and the nature, scope, and impact of the proposed change. People facing change may experience a whole series of negative emotions such as anger, denial, frustration, or simply acceptance and resignation. All of these feelings need to be overcome when working toward committed and enthusiastic change implementation. In order to create change in a positive and lasting way, these perceptions cannot be ignored however difficult they may be. An important aspect of change management must be to involve staff at all levels, including everyone in defining the nature of the change required and the subsequent processes, not simply imposing change.

KEY CONCEPTS

There is an extensive and complex literature on the management and leadership of change and the challenges it produces.[3, 4, 5, 6, 7, 8, 9, 10, 11] In Chapter 7 of the first book in this series, *Managing and Leading in the Allied Health Professions*,[12] Christina Pond also provides a detailed analysis and discussion of leadership, which is an important adjunct to this and a later chapter in this volume on care pathways.

NHS management and organisational structures have been the subject of radical and constant change since the 1974 structural reorganisation[13] and the pace of 'reform' now seems to increase on an almost daily basis. Hooper and Potter[14] suggest that there are 'five key drivers' for change that, when combined with accurate timing—implementing change before a peak in performance is reached—allow latent energy from the previous change cycle to be used while still at the experimental stage of the new cycle. Hooper and Potter[8] stress the

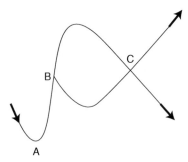

Figure 12.1 Learning dip and sigmoid curve

importance of leadership in maintaining the momentum of change linking this with the 'sigmoid curve'—shown in Figure 12.1—originally expounded by Charles Handy.[6] The sigmoid 'S'-shaped curve represents the life cycle of an individual or an organisation, which always waxes and then wanes. When starting a change project, there is an initial learning 'dip' before progress is quickly made. It is important to start the second curve at point 'A' before the peak, harnessing the latent energy of experience from the old curve while still at the experimental stage.

Burnes[15] cites three schools of thought:

1 **The individual perspective school:** supporters of this theory include the behaviourists who believe that behaviour results from an individual's interaction with his or her environment and the Gestalt-Field psychologists, who argue that an individual's behaviour is the product of behaviour and reason.

2 **The group dynamic school**: this school has the longest history; its emphasis is about bringing organisational change through teams or work groups rather than individuals. The rationale is that because organisations work in groups, individual behaviour must be seen, modified, or changed in light of groups' prevailing practices, postulating that group behaviour is an intricate set of symbolic interactions and forces that affect group structure and modify individual behaviours. The group brings about tensions that put pressures on its members.

3 **The open systems school**: the primary reference for this school is the organisation in its entirety. It suggests that any change to one part of the organisation will have an impact on all the other parts due to interconnected sub-systems and in turn an effect on performance. However, the organisation is not seen in isolation and is open to—and interacts with—the external environment as well as being open internally to the other sub-systems in the organisation. The objective of this approach is to structure the functions of the business in a manner that clearly defines lines of coordination and interdependence, emphasising achieving synergy rather than optimising performance of any one individual part.

In their discussion of the importance of managing change and how to handle the resultant anxiety that is associated with change, Obholzer and Roberts[16] emphasise the importance of understanding the different aspects of anxiety and its origins. Baker and Perkins[17] in their study of healthcare practitioners commented that change needs to be planned and managed, since the effective operation of a complex service is dependent on the goodwill, competence, and cooperation of its staff—change, they assert, can also threaten the efficiency of an organisation.

Pettigrew, Ferlie, and McKee[18] in their study of a variety of NHS changes proposed the concept of 'receptive' and 'non-receptive' contexts for change. Schon[19] argued that there is a 'conservative dynamic' within most organisations that strives to resist change; the positive side of this is the stability that is provided during times when change is not taking place.

Successful change according to Lewin[20] requires the 'unfreezing' of current attitudes, systems, and behaviours. He proposed that a programme of planned change and improved performance incorporates a three-phase process:

1 *Unfreezing*—reducing the forces that maintain the status quo; recognising the need for change and improvement to take place
2 *Transition*—the development of new attitudes or behaviours and implementation of the change
3 *Refreezing*—stabilising the change at the new level and supporting mechanisms in place to reinforce the change.

Burnes[3] set out a further range of change initiatives, including Total Quality Management (TQM) and Business Process Re-engineering (BPR). He concluded that change programmes were not guaranteed to succeed, but that the theory and practice of change management were an 'essential requisite for survival'.

CULTURE

A study of the concepts of attitudes and behaviours linked to management within an organisation introduces the concept of 'culture'. Schein[21] suggests that culture evolves as a complex outcome of external pressure, internal potential, critical events, and chance and proposed that cultural understanding is essential for leaders. Organisational culture—an important aspect that is often overlooked—warrants attention in change management processes. He proposed that culture and leadership are two sides of the same coin and could not be understood on their own, suggesting that the only thing of real importance that leaders do is to create and manage culture. Also he asserts that culture is in a sense a learned product of group experience and is to be found only when there is a definable group with a significant history. Therefore, according to Schein, a new group would have had no culture at the beginning, as it had no history. He suggests that culture evolves as a complex outcome of external pressures, internal potential, critical events, and chance.

Handy[22] had a different perspective, suggesting the four dominant cultures of:

1 club
2 role
3 task
4 person.

Schneider and Barsoux[23] discuss the interdependency between culture and structure. They commented on the different management styles adopted in Latin managers—who like formal structures and power division—whereas cultural styles and power division are adopted by Nordic and Anglo managers who believe that the world is too complex to be able to clearly define roles and functions. They concluded that effectively transferring management structures and processes rely on the ability to recognise inherent assumptions and compare with cultural assumptions.

The NHS has many cultures, including an overall public sector culture, sub-cultures at individual organisational levels, profession or occupational group subcultures, and teams. The importance of 'identity' and 'belonging' need to be acknowledged when introducing management reorganisation as lack of awareness of the importance of culture may be detrimental to the success of change management. Cultural changes take longer to accomplish than organisational restructuring, but an understanding of culture will help to facilitate effective change programmes.

LEADERSHIP

A clear understanding of leadership skills and techniques is essential for the success of any change management project.[12] The role and personality of a leader may be seen as the critical determinant of change management. Kotter[24] estimated that successful leadership—rather than management—is responsible for a high percentage of successful change. Handy[7] also suggests that leadership theory falls into categories of:

- trait
- style
- contingency.

Bennis and Nannus[10] have suggested that leadership has three main aspects:

1 commitment
2 complexity
3 credibility.

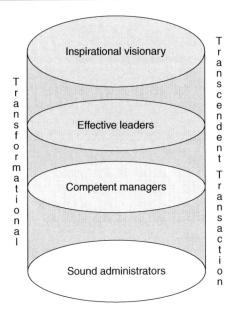

Figure 12.2 A hierarchy of leadership

Leadership vision was discussed by Wesley and Mintzberg[25] who proposed that most authors agree with the assertion that leadership vision can be broken into three stages of: envisioning, communicating effectively with followers, and empowering. Hooper and Potter[14] draw together concepts of transactional, transformational, and transcendent leadership, detailing the change from command and control leadership, through to empowerment. This theory has developed changes and evolution in leadership style.

Potter describes three levels of leadership: team, operational and strategic[26] other authors also suggest that leadership concepts are subdivided into three levels using a variety of terminologies, there is a degree of consensus surrounding many of the theories of leadership introducing the human relations aspect of change.

The concept of emotional intelligence was introduced by Daniel Goleman,[12, 27, 28] describing this as the ability to manage ourselves and our relationships effectively, with the four fundamental capabilities of:
1   self-awareness
2   self-management
3   social awareness
4   social skill.

Mastery of these areas, he argued, could enable the leader to choose the leadership style required for any given situation, including when undertaking change management.

TEAMS

There are many theories relating to team working. The difference between teams that perform well and others that do not is a subject that is often accorded too little attention in the context of management and leadership of change. Part of the problem might be that 'team' is a word and concept familiar to everyone in a wide range of contexts.

Team working and leadership are discussed in detail by Katzenback and Smith,[29] who emphasise the need for 'team purposing' when working collectively. They suggest that teams and good performance are inextricably linked. Their research shows that it is basic discipline that enables teams to work. Teams and good performance are inseparable, they argue; you can't have one without the other. Teamwork encompasses a set of values that encourage listening and responding constructively to views expressed by others.

However, good performance can be attributed to other factors. There is a distinct difference between a group of people brought together as a 'team' and a group that has a common vision and purpose. The latter produces individual efforts and 'collective work products', i.e. more than the sum of the individual contributors. The core is common commitment, which is only seen by a purposing team.[29]

Hirshhorn[30] highlights the damaging effect of interpersonal conflict that can occur within teams, making them dysfunctional.

MODELS, TECHNIQUES, AND APPROACHES FOR CHANGE MANAGEMENT

The management and leadership of change are both an imprecise science and art. However, there is a large, extensive evidence base from which to draw, including a wide range of theories and models—old and new—that might be applied to differing circumstances.

Before moving on to present our own 'Framework for the Management of Change', a brief overview of a few examples of the possible models, techniques, and approaches in this complex area may be useful to refer to. However, this review is far from exhaustive, as Figure 12.3 adapted from Iles and Sutherland[5]—which lists some examples—shows. It is intended to be useful to facilitate further exploration and for reference:

We set out below a selection of examples of various approaches that might be helpful in a variety of change management circumstances. These outlines are not intended as a 'how to do it' guide but as an indication of the range of models methodologies and techniques available.

Change process steps. Bristow *et al.*[31] outlined a process through which change development could be achieved.

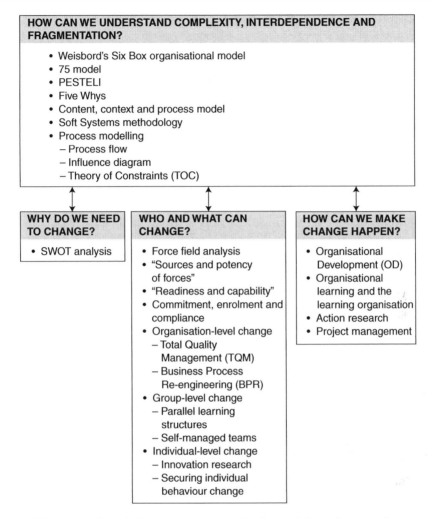

HOW CAN WE UNDERSTAND COMPLEXITY, INTERDEPENDENCE AND FRAGMENTATION?

- Weisbord's Six Box organisational model
- 75 model
- PESTELI
- Five Whys
- Content, context and process model
- Soft Systems methodology
- Process modelling
  - Process flow
  - Influence diagram
  - Theory of Constraints (TOC)

WHY DO WE NEED TO CHANGE?

- SWOT analysis

WHO AND WHAT CAN CHANGE?

- Force field analysis
- "Sources and potency of forces"
- "Readiness and capability"
- Commitment, enrolment and compliance
- Organisation-level change
  - Total Quality Management (TQM)
  - Business Process Re-engineering (BPR)
- Group-level change
  - Parallel learning structures
  - Self-managed teams
- Individual-level change
  - Innovation research
  - Securing individual behaviour change

HOW CAN WE MAKE CHANGE HAPPEN?

- Organisational Development (OD)
- Organisational learning and the learning organisation
- Action research
- Project management

Figure 12.3 An overview of change management tools, models, and approaches.

Box 12.1 Processes for development
- Recognise need for change.
- Seek help as required.
- Diagnose problem.
- Decide direction of change.
- Develop change plan.
- Evaluate and review.
- Continue cycle of development.

Table 12.1 Seven phases to social change intervention

Phase	Action
1 Develop the need for change	Begin unfreezing with problem awareness on the part of one or more managers/leaders
2 Establish the change relationship	Preliminary exploration between 'Change Agent' and client
3 Diagnose the planned system's problem	Collaborative data collection and analysis between Change Agent and client system
4 Examine alternatives and action goals	Stage change by determining action strategies and plans
5 Implement actions	Change activities and obtain feedback about results
6 Generalise and stabilise the change	Provide reinforcement to ensure workable changes are retained without backsliding
7 Evaluate and terminate 'Change Agent' relationship	Develop mechanisms for ongoing internal adjustment

Seven phases to social change intervention using an external 'Change Agent'. In this example, an external 'Change Agent' is brought into the organisation to facilitate the change process.[32] The 'client' is the 'host' organisation. Generally, change programmes are managed internally within the organisation without input from external sources.

Eight-Stage process of change. Wesley and Mintzberg[25] proposed an 'eight-stage' process of change.

Box 12.2 Eight-stage process of change
1 Establishing a sense of urgency.
2 Creating the guiding coalition.
3 Developing vision and strategy.
4 Communicating the change vision.
5 Empowering employees for broad-based action.
6 Generating short-term 'wins'.
7 Consolidating gains and producing more change.
8 Anchoring new approaches in the culture.

Change curve—reactions to change. The 'change curve' (Figure 12.4) represents the personal transitions and emotions a person tends to go through as they work through the change process. The reactions and responses generally follow a

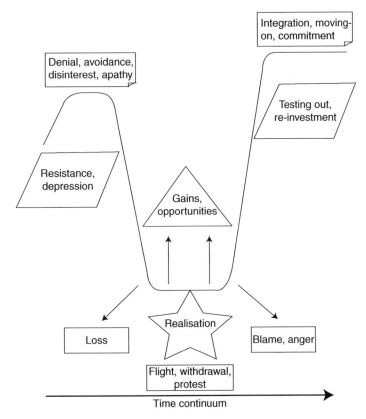

Figure 12.4 Reactions to change

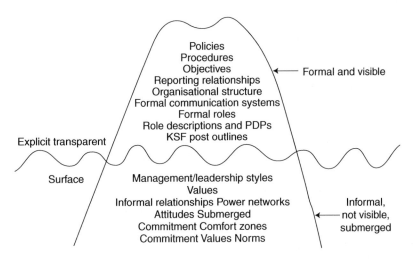

Figure 12.5 Iceberg process

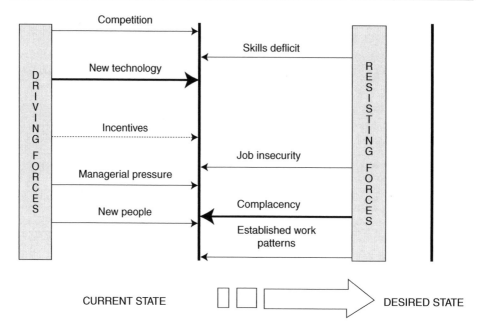

Figure 12.6 Force field analysis

particular pattern. The challenges for managers are to get the systems, process, and structures right and also, importantly, to help and support staff through the change process.

Iceberg process. The flow of tasks involved in implementing change is very often impeded by the underlying, submerged issues and behaviours. The barriers or resistance may have little to do with the rationale of the task being undertaken and everything to do with the feelings and relationships surrounding the task.

Therefore, awareness of the process is in itself not enough; the process has to be consciously managed and lead.

Force field analysis. The diagnostic technique of 'force field analysis' is used as a method of looking at variables involved in determining whether change will occur. It is based on the idea of 'forces' relating to perceptions about particular factors and their influences. Driving forces are those that 'push' in a particular direction, initiating change or keeping it going while restraining forces are acting to decrease the driving force or restraining it. It is a dynamic system approach to change and sees all situations as temporary and potentially changeable. At any given moment, a field of forces is acting on an event or problem. The approach involves identifying the forces and seeking to change their direction or strength.

PDSA analysis. During the 1930s, the PDSA cycle was developed as a model for process improvement in the context of change. It has been used ever since and was much vaunted by the NHS Modernisation Agency and is widely used as one of the techniques available in the management and leadership of change processes. The model illustrates the four phases of the PDSA cycle—plan, do, study, act—that may be used as part of improving a process or processes.

The phases of the PDSA cycle are:

- **plan** what you are going to do after gathering evidence of the nature and size of the problem
- **do** it, preferably on a small scale first
- **study** the results to ascertain whether a plan works
- **act** on the results, and if the plan was successful, standardise on the new way of working; if not successful, try an alternative.

See Chapter 14 of this volume on development of care pathways.

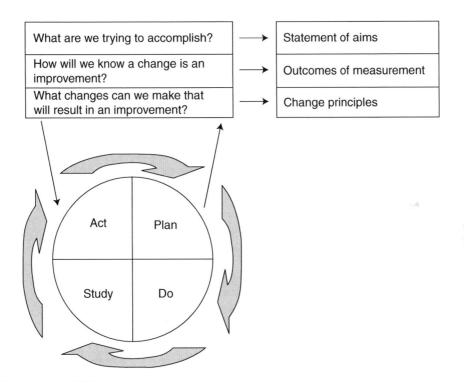

Figure 12.7 PDSA cycle

SWOT analysis

Subject of S.W.O.T. Analysis here; define the subject of the analysis here

Strengths
Advantages of proposition
Workforce
Capabilities
Competitive advantages
Unique selling points
Resources, assets
Experience, knowledge, data
Financial reserves likely returns
Marketing–reach, distribution,
    awareness
Innovative aspects
Location and geographical
Price, value, quality
Accreditations, qualifications
Processes, systems, IT,
    communications
Cultural, attitudinal, behavioural
Management and succession

Weaknesses
Disadvantages of proposition
Gaps in capabilities
Lack of competitive strength
Reputation, presence and reach
Financial
known vulnerabilities
Timescales, deadlines and
    pressures
Cost
Continuity
Effects on core activities,
    distraction
Reliability of data, plan
    predictability
Morale, commitment, leadership
Accreditations
Processes and systems
Management issues and succession

Opportunities
Market development
Competitors' vulnerabilities
Lifestyle trends
Technology development,
    innovation
Wider influences
New markets-vertical, horizontal
Niche target markets
Geographical
New unique selling points
Business developments
Information and research
Partnerships
Volumes, economies

Threats
Political effects
Legislative effects
Environmental effects
IT developments
Competitor intentions
Market demand
New technologies, services, ideas
Vital contracts and partners
Sustaining internal capabilities
Obstacles faced
Insurmountable weaknesses
Loss of key staff
Sustainable financial backing
Resistance to change
Home economy

Figure 12.8 SWOT analysis

PEST analysis

Insert subject for P.E.S.T. analysis–business, proposition...

Political	**Economic**
Environmental issues	Economic situation and trends
Current legislation	Market trends
Future legislation	Customer/end-user drivers
European/international legislation	
Regulatory bodies and processes	
Government policies	
Government term and change	
Funding, grants and initiatives	
Home and international lobbying/	
pressure groups	

Social	**Technological**
Lifestyle trends	Competing technology development
Demographics	Research funding
Consumer attitudes and opinions	Associated/dependent technologies
Media views	Replacement technology/solutions
Law changes affecting social factors	Maturity of technology
Brand, technology image	Capacity
Major events and influences	Information and communications
Role models	Technology legislations
Access	Innovation potential
Ethnic/religious factors	
Advertising and publicity	
Ethical issues	

Figure 12.9 PEST analysis

COMMUNICATING CHANGE

Change programmes sometimes fail and should not rely on 'Big Bang' announcements to persuade staff to 'fall in line'; this method is never advisable, leading to unsustainable change. Existing communication channels may be inadequate to report progress, particularly with a substantial change programme. When staff do not receive the information they need, they may turn to the 'grapevine'; the challenge for managers is to ensure that communication is timely, accurate, and all-inclusive.

Saunders[33] reports a study that shows:

- 20% of an organisation's employees tend to support change from the outset
- 50% are 'fence sitters'
- 30% are 'resistors' whom nothing can sway.

Communication strategy should therefore be initially aimed at the 70% of supporters and 'fence sitters'.

Box 12.3 Communication strategy
- Be specific about the change—staff should see the change programme as a tangible goal at organisational or departmental level, for example, reduce the length of stay by three days.
- Explain—to avoid staff feeling left in the dark about the reasons why change is required. Managers may have studied in depth the reasons why, but these need communicating to staff.
- Let staff know the scope of the change—even when the news is not good. Rumours can be worse than reality; it is better to inform staff if changes to staff numbers or redundancies are needed.
- Ensure two-way communication—meeting with staff to listen to their views as well as to inform is vital to offer explanation but also to gather ideas from the 'front line'.
- Be repetitive about the change plans and actions—if staff hear the message several times, they will be clear about the message, the reasons for change, and the consequences of not addressing the problem.
- Use pictures and graphs—many people retain information best if they see it visually.
- Use multiple methods for communication—posters, flyers, e-mails, letters, videos in staff canteens, and Web-based information as well as the invaluable one-to-one or group meetings are all avenues to be explored to get key messages across to staff and stakeholders.
- Gain middle-manager support—use this tier of management effectively; they are key to implementing the programme and have significant influence in the organisation.
- Offer training—training to build up new skills will support staff who need to be confident that the new system will work; equipped with new skills, they will support the process.
- Model the changes yourself—it is important that managers embrace the change themselves—rather than just expect staff to change—and words and actions need to be consistent with the change strategy.

CHANGE LEADERSHIP

Managers need to develop a range of leadership competencies to ensure the success of change programmes.

HOW TO OVERCOME 'CHANGE FATIGUE'

All organisational change involves three phases:[34]
- initial recognition and preparation; design of a response to set goals
- implementation of changes; the period of often 'hard-won' change
- consolidation period; when the organisation reviews and adjusts.

Table 12.2 Change leadership

	Organisational change agenda	*Leadership competency profile*
Executing strategy	• Customer focus • Innovate and be creative • Outcome focus	• Focus on client value; cultivate relationships • Drive innovation • Deliver results consistently
Creating value	• Mission, vision, values • Creativity and alignment Communicate openly • Teamwork • Sustainable change	• Strategy shaping • Building commitment • Team building and development • Develop organisational learning

The three phases are not linear and the second one is often considered to be the most difficult, where resistors need to be brought 'on board'. Change programmes may fail for two main reasons:

1 poor design—where underlying processes, for example, the way resources are allocated, or waiting for the ideal IT solution and not addressing specific behavioural problems
2 poor communication—change leaders must be prepared to communicate the same message at least six times—to ensure the message is heard by all. Staff must hear the arguments for and against the change options; they also need to hear that the organisation will support them through the change process.

The change leader should avoid trying to detail in advance the precise shape of the future—as failure to reach this precision can be virtually guaranteed and this can be demoralising. A better tactic is to outline the goals at the outset and improvise as the change project develops.

The key to substantive improvement lies in creating an environment in which change becomes part of the culture being continual, gradual, and low level. Change is more effective and sustainable if it relies on staff motivation rather than directives downwards from the top of the organisation.

Table 12.3 Leading change—why transformation efforts fail

Error 1	Not establishing a great enough sense of urgency
Error 2	Not creating a powerful enough guiding coalition
Error 3	Lacking a vision
Error 4	Undercommunicating the vision by a factor of 10
Error 5	Not removing obstacles to the new vision
Error 6	Not systematically planning for and creating short-term wins
Error 7	Declaring victory too soon
Error 8	Not anchoring changes in the organisation's culture

CRITICAL MISTAKES AND ERRORS

In his article 'Why Transformation Efforts Fail', Kotter[35] identifies eight possible 'critical mistakes-errors' and why 'hard-won' gains may be negated:

KEY FACTORS IN EFFECTIVE CHANGE MANAGEMENT

Paton and McCalman[4] identified 10 key factors in effective change management based on:

- innovative responses to triggers for change
- holistic solutions
- visionary leadership
- committed support.

The 10 factors—they argue—must be addressed and actioned if change is to be effectively managed. By ensuring that these factors have been considered before initiating change, the 'problem owner' and associated Change Agents will be in a position to confidently manage the process of transition.

A summary of the 10 factors is shown in Table 12.4.

Table 12.4 Change management factors

1 Change is all-pervasive	Any change process is likely to have an impact greater than the sum of its parts. 'A holistic view must be taken to ensure that the full impact is understood'; look at the whole picture.
2 Effective change needs active senior management support	It is vital that senior managers support the change process.
3 Change is a multidisciplinary activity	Most successful changes are brought about through teamwork. No one person is a 'change island', and recognition of the multidisciplinary nature of change is important in the sequence of achieving transformation.
4 Change is about people	People are the most important assets within an organisation or service; the team must be involved in the process from the outset, active participation is vital to gain commitment and 'ownership' of the change process. Change management is about people management and leadership. Essential elements are: • openness • good communication • involvement.
5 Change is about success	Dinosaur organisations and services become extinct through failure to adapt to the changing environment—it is important to set goals for success that can be achieved and be seen to be deliverable.

Table 12.4 Change management factors (*Continued*)

6 Change is a perpetual process	Something else always comes along to further impact: 'How do we explain change that was successful? How do we explain change that never seemed to get going? How can we explain the change project that started off well, but seemed to fade away after a couple of years? The answers seem to lie in the attention and resources devoted to managing change as a perpetual process … change is about identifying triggers, seeking vision, recruiting converts to the vision, and maintaining and renewing the need for change management action is necessary on all these fronts'.[4]
7 Effective change requires competent Change Agents	Change Agents (managers, leaders, and teams) require appropriate skills, knowledge, and position; a wide range of competencies is necessary for the achievement of successful outcomes. 'People skills' are essential and often difficult competencies to acquire.
8 There is no one best way or methodology	It is important not to take a 'blinkered' or 'singular' approach; what works for one change situation may not be appropriate to another.
9 Change is about 'ownership'	It is important that all involved feel 'ownership' and that the process is 'owned' by the problem owners, the Change Agents—managers, leaders, and teams—and those affected by the change. It is also essential that the management team feel that they are responsible for the successful implementation of the change. This implies the concept of the management team moving from control to commitment and support. When people are coerced or manoeuvred into change situations by threat or crisis, the result is at best indifference and at worst resistance. When people 'own' the change process and feel that it offers opportunities, they are much more likely to be committed to achieving a successful outcome.
10 Change is about fun, challenge, and opportunity	'When faced with a challenge, most individuals respond positively. 'We use "fun", in this instance, to denote an attitude of mind … throughout the seriousness of it all—the drive for performance, the need to maintain competitive edge, the desire for better, more effective organisation—there is also a need to show a human face'.[4]

KEY BEHAVIOURS AND SUCCESS FACTORS

We have shown that there are many possible approaches, models, techniques, and methodologies for bringing about successful change and there are no 'one only solution' for moving from the current to a newly desired situation. However, we believe that there are a number of key behaviours and success factors that can usefully be identified to help make the process positive and that we have incorporated into our 'Framework for the Management of Change', including for example:

Table 12.5 Key behaviours and success factors

Behaviours	Success factors
Proactivity	A long-term perspective
Inclusiveness, people involvement at all levels and across the whole team	Striving to achieve short- as well as long-term 'wins'
Flexibility	Development of vision and goals
Innovation	Using measures of success
Learning organisation/service	Benchmarking
Maintain focus	Maintain focus
Ability to use a variety of management styles	Use of appropriate knowledge and skills from within the team
Maintain calmness in challenging situation	Understanding the context
Integrity	Strategic-level support
Honesty	Management support
Openness	Keep it simple at all times; overcomplexity loses time and context
Coaching	Manage and lead with a clearly defined and explicit set of organisational/service values
Excellent communication	Identification and implementation of appropriate training/education
Celebration of success	Celebration of success

These suggestions are not in specific priority order and are not all-inclusive.

FRAMEWORK FOR THE MANAGEMENT OF CHANGE

An essential part of every manager's work is the management of change. There are a multitude of different approaches and methods that can be taken to facilitate successful outcomes. We have developed a 'Framework for the Management of Change' that builds on theoretical evidence, combining this with our practical experience in this field of management. The framework is not proposed as a 'one only way of doing it' or 'recipe', but rather a template that indicates the necessary consideration and steps to be taken at each phase of the change process. The framework has been tested in a number of situations and has been shown to facilitate successful and sustainable service improvement.

We developed the framework collaboratively with a view to facilitating specific change management projects. We wanted to incorporate established theory and practice into a simple methodology that could be adopted in a wide range of change situations and also support others in managing and leading change management processes.

Box 12.4 Framework for the management of change

1   Moving from the current to the desired situation
   - Identify 'triggers' for change
   - Managerial imperatives
   - Establish project group
   - Shared vision, objectives, and critical success factors

2   Essential actions
   - Data and information
   - Timing
   - Setting the direction
   - Staff participation at all levels
   - Negotiation with stakeholders
   - Specification phase
   - Implementation
   - Determine evaluation parameters

3   Skills for success
   - Management:
      i   responsibility, accountability, authority
      ii   commitment
      iii   strategic thinking
      iv   creativity
      v   negotiating and influencing skills
      vi   resources
      vii   political awareness
      viii team working.
   - Leadership:
      i   clear vision and focus
      ii   enthusiasm and commitment
      iii   communication
      iv   ability to challenge 'comfort zones'
      v   empowerment of staff at all levels
      vi   ownership
      vii   create alignment.

4   Evaluation
   - Completion within time scale
   - Completion within resources
   - Success criteria
   - Training
   - Service user feedback
   - Staff feedback

- Stakeholder feedback
- Adjust and reevaluate
5 Learning points
  - Understanding the context
  - Constraints and barriers
  - Clear vision of desired situation
  - Importance of people
  - Variety of management styles
  - Communication—timely, frequent, open
  - Infrastructure—organisational support
  - Resilience

CASE STUDY 'CHOICE APPOINTMENTS'

'Choice appointments' is an innovative appointment system for outpatient physiotherapy and other AHPservices.

In 2003, an innovative system for outpatient physiotherapy appointments was introduced at Eastbourne District General Hospital. This service redesign initiative was intended to improve patient choice and control over the intervention and treatment programmes, decrease 'did not attends' (DNAs) and 'unable to attends', decrease waiting times, decrease the number of complaints about long waiting times, and maximise clinical outcomes.

The system—designed in accord with our 'Framework for the Management of Change'—enables routine physiotherapy musculoskeletal outpatients to book same-day appointments at times of their choice for both first appointments and follow-ups.

MOVING FROM THE CURRENT TO THE DESIRED SITUATION
Triggers for change

Musculoskeletal problems represent around 30% of all GP consultations and account for between 30% and 35% of physiotherapy services. Referral sources include GPs, consultants and their teams, self-referral, and a range of other disciplines and professions.

The triggers for change included the volume of DNAs that on the departmental audit figures for the previous three years indicated a level of 11.3% per annum, significant wasted resources. Waiting times for non-urgent referrals were around 14 weeks and there were several complaints per month relating to long waiting times for outpatient physiotherapy. There was a desire to offer patients more choice about the days and times of their attendance and give more control over the quantity of intervention to patients. A further assumption was that clinical outcomes would be further improved if interventions were quicker, rather than patients having to wait up to 14 weeks for first appointments—prompt intervention is clinically effective and patients want to get back to full function as quickly as possible.

Managerial imperatives

To redesign the outpatient appointment system with the objective of eliminating DNAs, cutting waiting times, decreasing complaints about waiting times, improving patient control and choice at no extra cost, and striving to provide a responsive service for referrers and to be well within the requirements of commissioners.

These objectives were also in line with the political imperatives of providing greater choice for service users, cutting waste, contributing to the speed of throughput to support Trust waiting list initiatives, and ensuring a responsive appointment booking system was in place—being 'in tune' with wider political agendas. It was also seen as important for the service to be well-positioned for new developments being introduced into the NHS such as Payment by Results, Practice-based Commissioning, Choose and Book, and so on.

Establish project group

The project group for this work was already in place; the group comprised the outpatiens physiotherapy team led by the outpatient physiotherapy manager—the team already met on a weekly basis and was augmented on an ad hoc basis as necessary to include other key staff such as the receptionist.

Shared vision, objectives, and critical success factors

Development of shared vision evolved over several meetings. The new system was unique and therefore had no template on which to build or experience on which to draw. The overall aim was to introduce a system by which patients could book first appointments and follow-ups by phone on the days and for the times they wished to attend, basing the system on a capacity planning methodology. The key objectives were to decrease DNAs, decrease waiting times, decrease complaints, improve patient satisfaction, offer greater choice and control to patients, ensure 'best quality possible' clinical outcomes, and meet managerial and political imperatives. The critical success factors would comprise these aims and objectives which would be used as audit parameters to assess the success, or otherwise, of the system.

ESSENTIAL ACTIONS
Data and information

Timely, accurate, and relevant data is required before the change process commences, as a background to underpin the development process. A wide range of data is required at all stages to facilitate management of the change project in all its aspects. Data collection, analysis, and interpretation are crucial to all management work and wherever possible this should be supported by appropriate computerised information systems. Meaningful information can then be shared within the team and outside it to facilitate the change management process.

Timing
Time scales were agreed within the team for implementation of the phases of development.

Setting the direction
The direction of the project was led by the outpatient physiotherapy manager who also oversaw the development of paperwork and IM&T systems support. The physiotherapy manager was given responsibility for liaising with GPs, consultants, and their teams and other interested parties.

Staff participation at all levels
The physiotherapy outpatient team was included at all stages of the development including reception staff, assistants, physiotherapists at all grades, clerical staff, the therapy services IM&T officer; patients and referrer's views were sought and represented by the outpatient physiotherapy manager. The head of therapy services supported the group and also acted as a liaison within the trust and outside.

Negotiation with stakeholders
Stakeholders were involved and informed by the physiotherapy manager and head of therapy services. A number of specific negotiations also took place throughout the course of the development, for example, with a telephone company for the provision of a phone system at favourable terms. Commissioners were also kept fully informed of the development.

Specification phase
The existing service had been fully reviewed in terms of measurement of DNAs, waiting times, and patient satisfaction, for example. It had not been possible to undertake any literature review as nothing could be found in the literature to support the development of this unique system. Following detailed discussion and work within the team and discussion with stakeholders, the physiotherapy manager committed the system—including the capacity planning—to paper. The paperwork also underwent a series of further changes as the system was further developed and evolved; there is no 'finish point' in a dynamic development such as this.

Implementation

Having completed the specification and all preceding stages, the system was implemented in late in 2003. This was the culmination of several months development work. However, the system continued through a further series of changes based on audit, feedback, and evaluation over a long period. Authority to implement the system was based within therapy services and 'outside' permissions were not necessary.

Determine evaluation parameters

Evaluation parameters were set and agreed to ensure that the change programme met the aims, objectives, direction, and vision. The parameters agreed were: measurement of DNA rates, waiting list monitoring, assessment and measurement of number and content of complaints, formal audits of patients' views and level of satisfaction or otherwise, formal audit of those patients who did not contact the physiotherapy department (having been referred), formal audit of clinical outcomes, and audits of referrer views and staff/team views.

All of these measures would be used to feed into further development to improve the system where necessary and to ensure that the change programme met the need of patients and all other interested parties.

SKILLS FOR SUCCESS
Management skills

The head of therapy services delegated responsibility for management and leadership of the change project to the outpatient physiotherapy manager who was accountable for the process. This included the delegation of authority to bring about the changes agreed within the team. The head of therapy services was fully committed to supporting the physiotherapy manager and his team through the process.

- *Strategic thinking skills* were essential to ensure that the overall vision and direction were maintained throughout.
- *Creativity* was required on the part of the whole team throughout the entire process; 'Choice Appointments' was a 'first' in the UK and a number of problem-solving techniques and innovative ways of thinking were essential to the success of the project. Too often the pressures of daily patient care provision, managerial, financial, and other important demands push managers into a reactive approach; however, the experience was that creativity and proactivity can flourish if carefully led.
- *Negotiating and influencing skills* were called upon throughout. For example, some team members were sceptical about the possible benefits of the new system and resistant to the idea of 'surrendering' more control over episodes of physiotherapy care to patients. It was necessary to negotiate with these team members and ensure that their views were actively listened to and incorporated to influence

views. There were also negotiations and influencing strategies to be used in discussion with GPs, commissioners, and consultants.

- *New resources* were not required for this project; however, the physiotherapy manager was able to negotiate funding for a telephone system from voluntary sources and persuade the providing company to supply this at a favourable price.
- *Political skills* were needed for a basic understanding of the micro and macro contexts for introduction of the system and it was necessary to exercise strategic political skills.
- *The management style* adopted ensured participation and team working, that all involved could participate fully in the development, and that their contributions were valued and important. A variety of management styles were employed in different situations, where for example, decisions needed to be formalised and adhered to, responsibility having to be taken and authority to implement various phases at agreed times. The ability to adopt appropriate management skills and styles in different circumstances is an important attribute of management. The achievement of 'ownership' and participation is dependent on well-managed and well-led team working.

Leadership skills

- *Clear vision* and focus on the desired outcomes situation and commitment to ensuring that the service was patient-centred and provided a tangible improvement in quality of care were essential elements.
- *Excellent communication* between all involved in the development and at all levels, all disciplines, groups, and stakeholders involved was essential. Good communication is more than a 'two-way process'; in order to achieve success, all those with an interest should be included: as a consequence, communication is multidirectional, not just two-way.
- *Change often challenges our comfort zones* and this project was no exception as not all participants were equally enthusiastic or committed at the outset. Leadership and management skill needs to be exercised in challenging 'comfort zones' in a positive way in order to give time for the success of the project to reinforce advantages and benefits and 'win people over'. The challenging of 'comfort zones' often needs to take place, but in a positive manner.
- *'Ownership'* of the project was ensured by full team participation in the development work that engaged all team members and thus empowered them in the redesign process.

EVALUATION

Implementation within the agreed timescale was achieved. 'Choice Appointments' was unique, encompassing a totally new appointments system and new ways of working—giving more control to patients. As such, the system needs ongoing

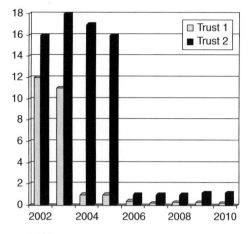

Figure 12.10 Percentage DNA

adjustments and further innovation in the light of experience and feedback from patients, staff, and other stakeholders. Examples of changes implemented later have been the introduction of new paperwork to support the system, improved use of IM&T, refined capacity planning, and so on.

The success criteria were met and exceeded.

*   DNAs were reduced from 11.3% per annum to less than 1% within the first three months, saving capacity of 11.3%—time wasting is eliminated—with the result that staff are able to spend more time with patients and effectively plan clinical-related work such as record keeping, team meetings, and in-service training. Importantly, capacity for taking more patients is increased.
*   Waiting times for non-urgent referrals were decreased from around 14–16 weeks to only a few days. During the last seven years, there were no complaints about waiting times.

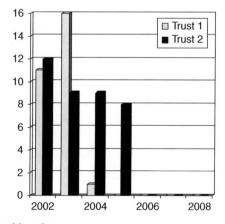

Figure 12.11 Routine waiting time

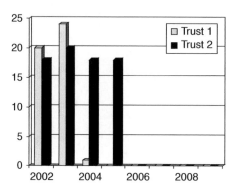

Figure 12.12 Waiting time complaints

Another trust adopted the system with similar results, reducing DNAs from 17% per annum to less than 1%, waiting time from 12–14 weeks to a few days, and liberating 22% greater capacity within the department. The bar charts in Figures 12.10, 12.11, and 12.12 illustrate these dramatic results for both services.

Formal audits have been undertaken in both services that indicate 94% patient satisfaction with the system (based on 100% questionnaire return, *see* Figures 12.13 and 12.14).

All these service improvement outcomes were achieved without any increase in resource input in financial terms, although time and effort were invested in setting up the system.

Further audits including clinical outcomes have been put in place to ensure that views and feedback from patients, staff, and stakeholders are incorporated into ongoing development.

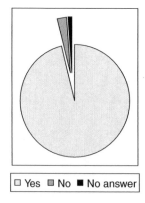

Figure 12.13 Was the information provided by the physiotherapy service appointment system clear?

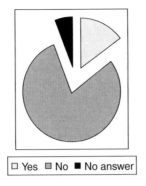

☐ Yes ▣ No ■ No answer

Figure 12.14 Would any other information have been useful?

LEARNING POINTS

In this case, as in all change management programmes, it is a dynamic environment in which the project is never fully completed, as there is a continuing process of audit and feedback together with constant change taking place within the organisation and wider health economy. It is therefore important that the system continues to develop in the light of the feedback, audit, and other environmental changes taking place. However, following implementation of the system and having achieved the main aims and objectives, a process of reflection took place to assist learning from the experience and to incorporate lessons into other developments taking place and for the future.

- An understanding of the context in which the work took place in all its aspects was important to aid the development, vision, direction, and implementation of the new system.
- Acknowledgement and understanding of constraints and barriers is essential so that strategies can be developed to overcome these; it is necessary to appreciate that it is not possible to improve or change all parameters surrounding the project.
- A clear vision of the desired situation—outcomes—helps cohesiveness of the team and ensures that everyone can be aware of, and sign up to, the overall aims and objectives.
- Involvement of people in the process from start to finish is crucial to success. All team members have important contributions that need to be listened to, understood and addressed, and incorporated. Thorough communication that is timely, in all directions, clear, open, and inclusive is essential. This will achieve 'ownership' and help to generate enthusiasm.
- Management support is essential at senior level to provide the multifaceted backup, ensure that the authority is delegated so that things can be made to happen, and that managers and leaders involved in the project have responsibility for achieving the desired outcomes and are held accountable appropriately for the development. Senior managers also need to ensure that all the necessary infrastructures are in place to support the development.

- Resilience is needed on the part of all involved because things do not always go well or according to plan. Sometimes it is necessary to rethink the strategy, try another way, or simply acknowledge and reject elements that do not give the positive answer envisaged.

CONCLUSIONS

- Sustainability: 'choice appointments' has been in place for almost a decade and has been highly acclaimed by patients. Audit of patients' views about the service gave very positive results on a 100% completion of the audit questionnaire by 355 consecutive patients over a six-week period.

The system fulfilled all the original aims and objectives and is popular with referrers.
- Nationally, other services have adopted the system en bloc or elements of it. Feedback has been positive with significant interest in the system.
- Approximately 800 people have attended courses led by the authors nationally and internationally on capacity and demand planning and the implementation of 'choice appointments'.
- At the Institute for Health Improvement European Forum (Prague), the system was acclaimed by the IHI president as an 'outstanding example of a Kano Type 2 project. Excellent for patient care and introduced at no extra financial cost'.

CONCLUSION–CHANGE MANAGEMENT

Change management describes a structured approach to transition. There are many roles and responsibilities for AHP managers in change management, from recognising trends in the macro as well as in the microenvironment; change is a fact of life and not an option. The speed of change has increased dramatically in the NHS and society generally in recent years.

The world may not be spinning faster, but mankind certainly is.[4]

In this chapter, we have shown that change management is not a distinct discipline with clearly defined and rigid boundaries, but that the theory and practice draws on a wide range of social science disciplines and traditions. The management of change has an extensive literature, being one of the most widely written about topics in the field of management. For this chapter, we have selected a few of the many approaches, methodologies, techniques, and models that we believe will be a useful guide for AHP managers.

We have also set out our own 'framework for the management of change' that is based on established change management theory and have presented a case study to demonstrate its practical application.

Change management cannot be seen in isolation, as there is always interaction with the external environment as well as with internal sub-systems within organisations. It is important that change management incorporates careful and thoughtful planning and sensitive introduction and implementation including real consultation with, and involvement of, the people affected by the change as well as those involved in the redesign and implementation process. Sometimes managers will need to support staff to overcome negative thinking—which may present obstacles to change—embodied in phrases such as 'we've always done it that way'. Strong resistance to change may be rooted in deeply conditioned or historically reinforced feelings and practices, and in this context, it is important that managers are aware of the various stages typically involved when change is imposed:

Box 12.5 Reactions to change

Denial–'This can't be real' or 'This is not happening'

Anger–'Why our team?' or 'How can they do this to us'?

Bargaining–'If I do this, you do that ...'

Depression or defeat–'This is going to happen'

Acceptance–move on

When change is forced on people, problems generally arise. Change must always be realistic, achievable, and measurable. Before embarking on change management projects, it is essential to answer the questions:
- what do we want to achieve with the proposed change?
- do we need outside help in bringing about the change?
- how and when will we know that the change has been successful?
- how will staff, the service, and organisation be affected by the change and how will they react?

It is important to remember that often the greatest insecurity for most staff is change itself; change may be disturbing and threatening. The manager has responsibility to facilitate and enable change, and the behaviour of managers is crucial to the success of the process; for example, some attitudes and behaviours can be counterproductive, such as the use of inappropriate language: 'We must change people's mindsets' or 'change people's attitudes'. Expressions such as these are likely to signal imposed change. In order to achieve positive outcomes, participation and involvement are essential with open, early, and fully inclusive communication.

As we have indicated there are a number of clearly definable principles involved in successful change management, including:
- always involve people and provide appropriate support
- understand where the organisation is at the moment—the current situation

- understand where you want to get to—the vision, desired situation
- understand when, why, and what the measures and monitoring procedures will be
- plan development in appropriate, measurable stages
- communicate, involve, listen, enable, and facilitate
- put relevant training programmes in place where necessary
- celebrate success
- evaluate, learn, and readjust
- do not decide on the end before you begin.

There are many challenges and opportunities for AHP managers in the NHS to manage and lead change and to become involved in this important area of management practice; a positive, informed, and systematic approach is essential for the achievement of successful outcomes.

REFERENCES
1. Heraclitus. In: *The Oxford Library of Words and Phrases. Vol. 1 Quotations.* Oxford: Oxford University Press; 1981.
2. Johnson S. Of the laws of ecclesiastical polity. In: *The Oxford Library of Words and Phrases. Vol. 1 Quotations.* Oxford: Oxford University Press; 1981.
3. Burnes B. *Managing Change—a strategic approach to organisational dynamics.* Harlow: Pearson Education Ltd; 2000.
4. Patton R, McCalman J. *Change Management—a Guide to Effective Implementation.* London: Sage Publications; 2000.
5. Iles V, Sutherland K. *Managing Change in the NHS. Organisational change—a review for healthcare managers, professionals and researchers.* NCC SDO; 2001. www.sdo. lshtm.ac.uk.
6. Handy C. *The Empty Raincoat.* London: Hutchinson; 1994.
7. Handy C. *Understanding Organisations.* London: Penguin Business Books; 1999.
8. Hooper A, Potter J. *The Business of Leadership; adding lasting value to your organisation.* Aldershot: Ashgate Publishing; 2002.
9. Mintzberg H, Quinn JB. *The Strategy Process; concepts, contexts and cases.* New Jersey: Prentice-Hall; 1988.
10. Bennis W, Nannus B. *Leaders: strategies for taking charge.* New York: Harper Business; 1997.
11. Mullins L. *Management and Organisational Behaviour.* Harlow: Pearson Education Ltd; 2002.
12. Pond C. Leadership in the Allied Health Professions. In: Jones R, Jenkins F, editors. *Allied Health Professions—essential guides. Managing and leading in the Allied Health Professions.* Oxford: Radcliffe Publishing Ltd; 2006.
13. Jones R, Jenkins F. *Allied Health Professions—essential guides. Managing and leading in the Allied Health Professions.* Oxford: Radcliffe Publishing Ltd; 2006.
14. Hooper A, Potter J. *Intelligent Leadership.* London: Random House; 2001.

15. Burnes B. *Managing Change—a strategic approach to organisational dynamics.* Harlow: Pearson Education Ltd; 1996.
16. Obholzer A, Roberts V. *The Unconscious at Work: individual and organisational stress in the human services.* Hove: Brunner Routledge; 2000.
17. Baker A, Perkins D. Managing People and Teams. In: Glynn J, Perkins D, editors. *Managing Healthcare.* Canterbury: Saunders; 1995.
18. Pettigrew F, McKee, L. *Shaping Strategic Change.* London: Sage; 1992.
19. Schon D. *Beyond the Stable State.* New York: Lawton; 1971.
20. Lewin K. Groups Decisions and Social Change. In: Swanson G, Newcomb TM, Hartley EL, editors. *Readings in Social Psychology.* New York: Holt, Rinehart and Winston; 1958.
21. Schein E. *Organisational Culture and Leadership.* San Francisco: Jossey-Bass; 1992.
22. Handy C. *The Gods of Management.* London; Random House: 1991.
23. Schneider S, Barsoux J. *Managing across Cultures.* Harlow: Pearson Education; 2003.
24. Kotter J. *Leading Change.* Boston, Harvard Business School; 1996.
25. Wesley F, Mintzberg H. Visionary leadership and strategic management. In: Henry J, Walker D. *Managing Innovation.* London: Sage; 1999.
26. Potter J. *Introducing the Human Relations Aspect of Change.* Exeter University: Centre for Leadership Studies; 2002.
27. Goleman D. *Emotional Intelligence—why it can matter more than IQ.* London: Bloomsbury Publishing; 1996.
28. Goleman D. Leadership that gets results. *Harvard Bus Rev.* 2000; Mar–Apr: 79–90.
29. Katzenbach J, Smith D. *The Wisdom of Teams.* Boston: Harvard Business School Press; 1993.
30. Hirshhorn L. *The Workplace Within.* Cambridge: Massachusetts Institute of Technology; 2000.
31. Thakur M, Bristow J, Carby K. An Introduction to organisational development. In: *Personnel in Change.* Institute of Personnel Management; 1978.
32. Lippit R, Watson J, Priestly B. *The Dynamics of Planned Change.* New York: Harcourt Brace Jovanovich; 1958.
33. Saunders R. Communicating Change. In: *Managing Change to Reduce Resistance.* Boston: Harvard Business School Press; 2005.
34. Garvin D. *Learning in Action: A guide to putting the learning organization to work.* Boston: Harvard Business School Press; 2000.
35. Kotter P. Leading Change—Why transformation efforts fail. *Harvard Bus Rev.* 1995; Mar–Apr: 59–67.

CHAPTER 13

Outcome measurement Matrix for AHP services

Robert Jones and Fiona Jenkins

INTRODUCTION

Outcome measurement is more important than ever before at this time of severe economic pressure and where patients are better informed and have increasingly high demands and expectations. Healthcare services need to be able to demonstrate effectiveness and efficiency—high clinicalvalue and value for money. Organisations are required to look very closely at how costs can be reduced or modified while at the same time having the objective of maintaining and improving quality of care. AHP service managers and leaders have to consider—in conjunction with others—whether all aspects of the services they provide are affordable. Healthcare commissioning and service planning must be based on clinical effectiveness and benefits realisation rather than on service provision founded on purely historical factors; in other words, if you do what you've always done, you'll get what you've always got. An essential part of the process is the use of patient outcome measures, including Patient Reported Outcome Measures (PROMS), which must be validated, consistent, and robust with assessment of the benefits of clinical interventions set against resource use.

In this chapter, we set out a methodology for outcome measurement recording and analysis. The objective is to facilitate evaluation of the end result of therapy interventions with individual patients and in aggregated form for groups of patients or specific populations and to present a system that is easy to use and applicable to many clinical situations and services. Outcome measurement—of which there are many techniques and approaches in use—is an essential element of the clinical process and necessary to the provision of efficient and clinically effective services. This Matrix system has been developed and used in an NHS Trust physiotherapy service[1] and has been further refined by the authors for use by other professional groups. Outcome measurement is of paramount importance in the context of the ongoing high intensity changes and reforms in healthcare service provision in the UK and worldwide; given the fiscal ice age, infinite demand, and finite resources. It is incumbent on providers of healthcare services to evaluate the outcomes of their interventions against resource use.

> 'These changes also reflect variations in values, attitudes, and expectations towards health and healthcare by health workers, patients, carers, health service managers, and officers in the Department of Health as well as government officials'.[2]

Variations on the basic system of measurement were devised to facilitate a straightforward methodology to enable collection, recording, and analysis of outcomes in a range of clinical services and interventions and these are presented here.

Outcomes are defined as:

> The end result of interventions with a client or a population in the short, medium, and long terms'[3]

In defining professional quality standards each service should:

> 'Reach towards defining quality in terms of outcome and health gain as well as in terms of process structure and inputs'.[4]

OUTCOME MEASURES FOR OUTPATIENT SERVICES

The system is based on measures of efficiency and effectiveness.

Effectiveness is calculated by measuring the extent to which the agreed goal or aims of a plan of treatment are achieved. When the patient is discharged from therapy, having completed an episode of treatment/care, they are asked to assess what improvement has taken place—compared with the situation at the outset—and to score this on a scale between one and seven. (Box 13.1)

Box 13.1 Effectiveness scoring

1 Worse
2 No change
3 Slight improvement (up to 25%)
4 Reasonable improvement (up to 50%)
5 Marked improvement (50% or more)
6 Great improvement (75% or more)
7 Completely better

The therapist also undertakes an assessment at the conclusion of the episode of care that compares with their initial assessment undertaken at the patient's first attendance. The therapist allocates a score between one and seven. The patient's score and the therapist's score are then added together and divided by two to give a combined score for clinical effectiveness. If the patient failed to complete the episode of treatment jointly agreed with the therapist, for whatever reason, a score of zero (0) is recorded.

An example of this is:

EFFECTIVENESS SCORE

Therapist's score based on parameters within the clinical assessment at the conclusion of the episode of care = 4 on the effectiveness scale, relative to scoring at the outset.

Patient assessment score = 6, relative to their assessment at the start of treatment, based on parameters such as severity of pain, activities of daily living, work, eating patterns, and communication skills.

The two scores are added together: 4 + 6 = 10. This score is then divided by 2, giving an overall combined patient and therapist score of 5 on the effectiveness scale. This is plotted on the effectiveness line, the horizontal axis of the Matrix. (Figure 13.1)

EFFICIENCY SCORE

Efficiency is defined as achieving maximum improvement using the least resources. For this, the number of treatment sessions in an episode of care are recorded on the vertical axis of the Matrix (Figure 13.1) and plotted against the measure.

The average number of physiotherapy treatments in an episode of care for patients with musculoskeletal problems in England in 2010 was 4.41.[5] This figure is therefore taken as the number of treatments representing the average on the vertical axis in this example. However, the average number of treatments will differ widely between different clinical services, types of intervention, and so on. The average might be set locally for a particular department, type of intervention, or clinical condition.

To illustrate the principle, this example shows effectiveness scored at 5.

The number of treatments in this episode of care is 3 (below the average of 4.41). This data is then plotted onto the outcome measurement Matrix (Figure 13.1).

OUTCOME MEASUREMENT MATRIX

The Matrix is represented by a square divided into four equal boxes—A, B, C, and D. These letters represent:

A: Less than the average number of treatments in the episode with high effectiveness score

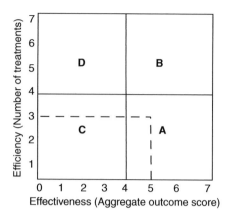

Figure 13.1 Outcome measurement Matrix—example 1

B: High level of effectiveness but number of treatments above the average

C: Low level of effectiveness and low number of treatments

D: Low effectiveness with high number of treatments

0: Represents failure to complete therapy episode, no effectiveness or efficiency outcome

Box **A** is the best outcome, as it indicates a lower than average number of treatments with a high level of effectiveness.

Box **B** indicates an acceptable but less desirable outcome with a satisfactory effectiveness measure but more than average number of treatments.

Box **C** represents an unacceptable outcome, as there is a poor response to therapy intervention although there is less than average number of treatments in the episode of care.

Box **D** is the poorest result, with poor effectiveness score and more than average number of treatments.

In this example, the effectiveness score of five is plotted onto the Matrix, and the efficiency score is calculated with three treatments for the episode being below the average (four treatments) and plotted onto the Matrix on the efficiency axis. The point at which the two dotted lines intersect in this example falls into Box A, and this letter represents the outcome measure, that is, an effective outcome with less than average therapy input. The overall outcome score is represented by the box letter in the Matrix, in this case, A.

If on the other hand, in another example, Figure 13.2, the effectiveness score is two and the efficiency score is six, the dotted lines will intersect on the Matrix in Box D, a poor effectiveness score and more than average number of treatments.

These results may be used to assess the outcome for individual patients or input into the computer for each patient and then aggregated to obtain service or population outcomes or outcomes for a particular condition or technique.

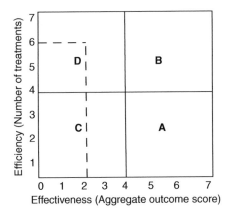

Figure 13.2 Outcome measurement Matrix—example 2

OUTCOME MEASURES: INPATIENT SERVICES

The basic principles for outcome measurement recording for inpatient therapy services are very similar to those for outpatients. However, it was necessary to modify the system in recognition of the different modes of working and other factors related to inpatient therapy care.

Effectiveness is taken as the extent to which the agreed goals or aims of a plan of treatment are achieved with the patient and therapist assessments based on a scale of one to seven, a similar method to that used in outpatient services. The average time for the care pathway in use is plotted halfway up the vertical—efficiency axis—this will be different for different care pathways, Figure 13.3. That is, a target time is set for goals to be achieved in the care pathway and this is represented as the average. This could be expressed in days or weeks. If the episode of care cannot be

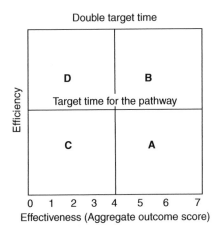

Figure 13.3 Outcome measurement Matrix—inpatients

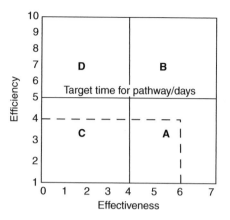

Figure 13.4 Outcome measurement Matrix–inpatients–example 3

completed, for example, if the patient is transferred elsewhere or the goal changes due to other clinical circumstances intervening, or the patient dies, a score of zero (0) is recorded.

Efficiency is to gain the maximum possible benefit using the least resources. The target time for the pathway is set and placed on the vertical axis. A point halfway up the vertical axis is marked, to represent the target time within the care pathway, Figure 13.3, the highest level on the vertical axis equals double the target time.

The effectiveness score is plotted against the target time on the grid.

Key:

0: Failed to complete treatment/goal/pathway changed

A: The optimum—good effect in less time than average on the pathway

B: Acceptable—satisfactory effect but over target time

C: Less than satisfactory outcome—as poor response to therapy interventions though less than average time in episode of care

D: The poorest outcome—poor effectiveness measure and extended time above average for pathway

This example (13.4) represents a pathway such as fractured neck of femur where the target completion and discharge might be five days. In this instance, the patient was discharged in four days and the effectiveness was six. This places the outcome in Box A; a good effect within less time than the target for the pathway.

OUTCOME MEASURES: COMMUNITY DOMICILIARY

In Community Domiciliary Therapy Services, the approach adopted for inpatient services is appropriate. Again, the effectiveness measure is a combination of the patient and therapist assessment and the efficiency factor is based on the time scale set out in the care pathway.

USING THE MATRIX FLEXIBLY

There are several hundred methodologies in use for the assessment and recording of outcomes, but it is not the purpose of this chapter to explore these. The examples set out in this chapter demonstrate just one method of recording the patient and clinician assessment of outcome relative to the resource use demonstrated through the number of treatments or interventions or time and illustrate how the Matrix can be used. The horizontal axis of the graph can be used to indicate a variety of clinical outcome measurement scores that can be set against the vertical axis, enabling the Matrix to be used for a variety of outcome measurement methodologies.

RECORDING OUTCOME MEASURES

The outcome of therapy interventions should be recorded in the patient's notes and also recorded on the computer information system so that the results can be analysed by teams and individual clinicians to assess effectiveness and efficiency and form a basis for comparison and learning to influence changes in practice, developments in interventions, and to form an essential element of the evidence base.

REFERENCES

1. Jones R. *An Investigation into the Development of a Computerised Information System for NHS Physiotherapy Services*. PhD thesis. England: University of Kent Business School; 2000.
2. Moore A. Outcome measurement in clinical practice. In Jones R, Jenkins F. *Managing Money, Measurement and Marketing in the Allied Health Professions*. Oxford: Radcliffe Publishing; 2010.
3. Ovretveit J. *Health Service Quality*. Oxford: Blackwell Science; 1992.
4. Long A, Dixon P, Hull R. The outcome agenda, contribution of the UK clearing house on health outcomes. *Qual. Healthcare*. 1993; 2(1): 49–52.
5. Chartered Society of Physiotherapy. *Physiotherapy Outpatient Waiting Time Survey 2010*. London: CSP; 2010.

CHAPTER 14

Care pathways and the Allied Health Professional

Fiona Jenkins and Robert Jones

THE LINK BETWEEN AHPS AND CARE PATHWAYS

AHPs provide healthcare in a wide variety of settings, for example, hospital inpatient, outpatient, domiciliary, occupational health, and schools. AHPs also work at different levels of authority ranging from undergraduate supervised practice through a range of autonomous clinical positions, expert and consultant practitioners, and managerial posts. Whatever the profession, the place of work or grade of post, all AHPs have a duty to ensure that they provide the best possible service, which in turn requires them to deliver evidence-based care. Care pathways have been upheld by Roy as:[1]

The key to unlocking the national agenda for improved services, increased responsibility, through clinical governance, and an easy route into the information superhighway.

The term 'integrated' tends to refer to a combined pathway of care and a multidisciplinary documentation recording system. This chapter focuses primarily on the care pathway, although reference will be made to the all-encompassing Integrated Care Pathway (ICP). The combination of high quality multidisciplinary intervention underpinned by evidence-based practice is best provided through the use of the care pathway approach. For AHPs, this can be translated to mean providing the best possible coordinated service for the patients by:

- streamlining the patient journey through health/social care
- doing the right things in the right order—the right patient at the right time and place, in the right way, with the right outcome
- clarifying role and responsibilities of the multidisciplinary team
- involving patients in their own care
- ensuring that there is attention to the patient's experience
- developing appropriate patient information.

Clinical guidelines are often better at focusing on diagnosis and interventions than they are at ensuring that care is organised and effectively managed. Although patients are unique individuals, they are often similar enough to warrant the development of guidelines based on evidence to improve both the coordination and the consistency of care. Historically, the major focus of care pathways was the treatment of surgical patients in acute hospitals. However, there has been subsequent development of pathways that provide care in a range of settings and by a wider multidisciplinary team. AHPs need to ensure that their interventions are coordinated with the rest of the health and social care teams—and that the patient is truly central to receiving the best care possible. One of the main challenges facing healthcare professionals and managers is the need to make the best use of limited resources, while providing high quality, timely, evidence-based practice.

Potential benefits from this approach often fail to be realised due to poor project planning and management.

People and perfect processes make a quality health service—a poor quality service results from a badly designed and operated process, not from lazy or incompetent healthcare workers.[2]

Care pathways are a way of encouraging the translation of national guidelines into local protocols and their subsequent translation into local practice as well as a method for systematic gathering of clinical data for audit purposes.[3] As AHPs are involved in a wide spectrum of healthcare and provide interventions in diverse settings, they are ideally placed to ensure that care pathways are used to provide the best care for patients and clients; they are equally well placed to help develop pathways themselves.

We have designed this chapter to provide a step-by-step guide to developing both the integrated and care pathway versions developed following practical experience of developing, implementing, and monitoring multidisciplinary pathways with reference to a theoretical base.

WHAT IS A CARE PATHWAY

A care pathway contains a number of different elements, including planning and implementation, followed by ongoing review. The equivalent to pathways in industry would be called by other names, possibly a combination of good practice, quality control, plus a large portion of ongoing quality improvement and design modification. In healthcare, a care pathway is viewed as a multidisciplinary outline of anticipated care. However, confusingly there is no single agreed definition of an ICP. A number of definitions have been in use since the late 1990s. Some confusion has been created because they all link ICPs directly to patient groupings or case types. A single ICP rarely covers the full span of a patient 'journey' for a particular condition; the patient's care plan is commonly built up from a group of pathways, each of which describe a component or phase of the care for example an admission or assessment phase, a set of interventions. and a discharge phase.

Definitions commonly quoted include:

1 the European Pathway Association:[4] care pathways are a methodology for the mutual decision making and organisation of care for a well-defined group of patients during a well-defined period. Defining characteristics of care pathways includes:
   - an explicit statement of the goals and key elements of care based on evidence, best practice, and patient expectations
   - the facilitation of the communication, coordination of roles, and sequencing the activities of the multidisciplinary care team, patients, and their relatives
   - the documentation, monitoring, and evaluation of variances and outcomes and the identification of the appropriate resources
   - the aim of a care pathway is to enhance the quality of care by improving patient outcomes, promoting patient safety, increasing patient satisfaction, and optimising the use of resources.

2 *Journal of Integrated Care:*[5] an Integrated Care Pathway determines locally agreed, multidisciplinary practice based on guidelines and evidence, where available, for a specific client group. It forms all or part of the clinical record, documents care given, and facilitates the evaluation of outcomes for continuous quality improvement.

3 Evidence-based medicine:[6] a care pathway can be defined as a structured multidisciplinary outline of anticipated care, placed in an appropriate time frame, to help a patient with a specific diagnosis or set of symptoms move through a continuum of care, receiving evidence-based care to maximise positive outcomes.

4 Wilson:[7] a multidisciplinary process of patient focused care that specifies key events, tests, and assessments, occurring in a timely fashion to produce the best prescribed outcomes, within the resources and activities available, for an appropriate episode of care.

All the definitions emphasise that care pathways bring together evidence-based multidisciplinary practice for a particular group of patients, to outline the optimum episode of care for all patients who have a specific condition or who are undergoing specific procedures.

The current most widely accepted definition in the UK has been developed by the National Pathways Association (NPA):[8]

Box 14.1 NPA definition of a care pathway

An ICP determines locally agreed, multidisciplinary practice based on guidelines and evidence where available, for a specific patient/client group. It forms all or part of the clinical record, documents the care given, and facilitates the evaluation of outcomes for continuous quality improvement.

ICPs also known as coordinated care pathways, care maps, or anticipated recovery plans are essentially task-oriented care plans that set out essential steps in the care of patients with a specific diagnosis or problem and describe the patient's intended clinical plan.[9, 10] They are also useful in understanding why care sometimes falls short of locally adopted standards and can be a useful tool in supporting clinical audit and further service improvement.

THE HISTORY AND SPREAD OF CARE PATHWAYS

Critical path and process mapping methodology was used in industry, particularly in the field of engineering from as early as the 1950s. In the 1980s, clinicians in the United States began to develop the pathway tool within 'managed care'; redefining the delivery of care and attempting to identify measurable outcomes. The focus was on the patient rather than the system, but needed to demonstrate efficient processes in order to fulfill the requirements of the insurance industry.

In the early 1990s, the NHS funded a patient-focused initiative to support organisational change, resulting in investigation and development of concepts such as pathways. In 1990, a team from the UK visited the United States to investigate the use of these pathways or 'Anticipated Recovery Pathways' as they were then called. As a result, 12 pilot sites for pathways were set up in northwest London in 1991–92. The West Midlands pathway development work commenced. By 1994, the Anticipated Recovery Pathway had evolved in the UK, care pathways were clinician led and driven, and had patients and locally agreed best practice at the centre of their focus.

In response to demand for coordinated care pathway user groups, the National Pathways User Group—renamed the National Pathway Association—was set up in 1994. The NeLH pathways database and the International Web Portal were launched in 2002 to enable the free sharing of ICPs across the UK and to provide care pathway user and developer forums for discussion and sharing of best practice and development skills and has since been included as part of by the NHS Evidence website.[11] Since 1992, care pathways have been developed and implemented across many healthcare settings in the UK—acute, community, primary, mental health, private, independent, and NHS.

ICPs are now used all around the world, including in the United States, Canada, New Zealand, Australia, Germany, Belgium, and the Netherlands.

WHY DEVELOP CARE PATHWAYS?

There are many good reasons for developing pathways to provide a structured framework for both existing practice and developments. They:
- ensure the provision of consistent high-quality care
- transfer evidence-based care into practice

- are patient-centred, inclusive, and clinically driven
- reduce unnecessary variation in practice
- reduce risk
- provide integration of care across organisational boundaries
- enable training/education and skills transfer
- are a tool for systematic action to facilitate continuous improvements in patient care
- provide evaluation of the impact of service redesign and improvement
- are a model to underpin many key local and national agendas simultaneously
- provide an opportunity to involve teams in service redesign.

The use of pathways can ensure the care process is better monitored and streamlined for the majority of people in a given patient or client population, providing patients with more consistent care and services by minimising variations in practice. As they are based partly on previous clinical cases, providers are better equipped to predict all aspects of the care process, including milestones, complications, and outcomes, and improve the quality of care provided to the next patient with the same condition.

Care pathways help ensure a high degree of efficiently delivered care for a defined population. Once a pathway has been put in place, key indicators are regularly monitored to assess effectiveness. This information is used for learning rather than to judge individual performance and helps target areas in need of improvement.

WHAT CARE PATHWAYS CONTAIN
- Algorithms defining the planned pathway within a time frame.
- Referral, transfer, and discharge guidance.
- Local and national standards.
- Evidence-based guidelines.
- Patient information.
- Information recording—this will make the care pathway a full ICP and will form all or part of the clinical record. For example, problem-orientated medical record or similar structured freehand text area:
  - a system of review—variance tracking
  - tests, charts, assessments, diagrams, letters, forms, information leaflets, satisfaction questionnaires, and so on
  - scales for measurement and outcomes of clinical effectiveness
  - 'space' to add activities or comments to a standard ICP to individualise care for a specific patient.

CARE PATHWAYS AND CLINICAL GOVERNANCE
Care pathways provide defined standards and stages along the patient's 'journey' and they help reduce unnecessary variations in care, which may compromise clinical

outcome. Pathways improve multidisciplinary and multi-agency collaboration and, importantly, empower patients and carers to be informed about and engaged in the care programme.

Many patients receive care that spans not only health organisation boundaries, but also partner sectors such as education and social services. Working with organisations that mostly adhere to different governance principles may cause lack of clarity about lines of accountability. The Audit Commission[12] believes that it is vital that there should be clarity between partners regarding purpose, roles, and responsibilities. The use of care pathways strengthens clinical governance procedures within organisations and across them.

THE AIM OF CARE PATHWAYS

Patients whose care is organised and managed through pathways should be given realistic information about their healthcare as well as the likely progression of treatment and care. Involving patients will engage them actively, encouraging questions about prognosis and future healthcare needs, improving their satisfaction with services, and reducing misunderstanding and complaints.

Box 14.2 The aims of care pathways
- Provide best evidenced-based care
- Facilitate translation of national directives into local practice
- Improve multidisciplinary and multi-agency communication
- Sustain and make equitable quality standards
- Reduce variance in practices
- Improve clinician/patient communication and satisfaction
- Identify research and development questions
- Involve team members in service development

From the initial easily definable care pathways of the 1990s that addressed single procedures, there was an evolution of pathways that embraced the more complex conditions and ones that encompass not only inpatient healthcare, but also community and multi-agency care. With input from people with the appropriate range of skills, care pathways can be developed to ensure that optimum care is provided in every setting.

The ways in which care pathways have been developed vary; some people feel they should reflect the desired outcomes rather than only the current practice, because focusing on current ways of working may lack the impetus for change. Pathways should incorporate the evidence base with what is possible to provide locally with the resources available.

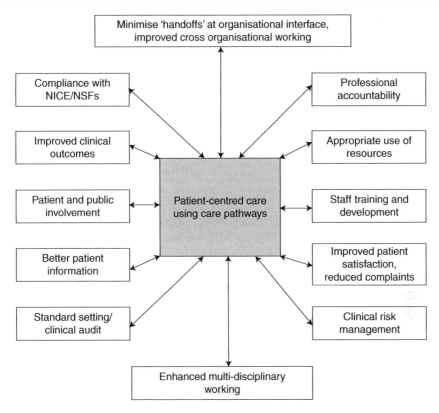

Figure 14.1 Integrated care pathways and clinical governance

Some practitioners consider the documentation recording system alone to be the care pathway. This is a misconception that must be addressed at the outset of development. The pathway is often depicted as an algorithm, showing various routes that the patient may take on the 'journey' through their healthcare programme—and is the template on which future care delivery will be based. The way in which documentation is used to support the pathway is one of the elements of developing a full ICP. Many organisations choose to develop referral guidelines or pathways that include algorithms but exclude unified documentation systems. In practice, both an algorithm of the care pathway and specifically developed documentation recording notes have been demonstrated to improve the quality of care, which requires best practice to be commissioned, provided, and evaluated.

The healthcare team is likely to benefit from the use of care pathways. Clinical teams are able to develop their team working skills, which have been shown to improve patient care.[12] Additionally, the relationship that exists between the professionals from different agencies involved in providing care for specific patient groups can be both defined and enhanced during the development of pathways. Each pathway should demonstrate commitment to:

• be patient-centred
• cross professional and organisational boundaries
• be evidence-based
• form a single shared record of care—where a full ICP is developed
• be audited and modified in light of this
• include feedback from users.

TEN PHASES TO DEVELOPING CARE PATHWAYS

We propose 10 phases for the development of a care pathway. There are several elements to be sequentially achieved in developing care pathways illustrated in Box 14.3. Each phase requires facilitation, management, decision-making, and team action.

Box 14.3 Ten phases to developing care pathways

1 Choose a clinical area.
2 Review the evidence.
3 Collect data and measure.
4 Review current practice including process mapping.
5 Identify key indicators.
6 Drafting the ICP.
7 Review and revise ICP draft.
8 Develop user version of care pathway.
9 Launch care pathways.
10 Monitor indicators, review, and amend.

Phase 1: choosing a clinical area

Selecting an important area of practice should be the first stage. A shared understanding of the organisation's strategic direction is essential, as is the commitment of senior management and clinical staff. A care pathway is, among other things, a change management tool and should be an integral part of the organisation's business and governance systems. The strategic 'vision' is imperative, which ensures that the whole team works toward a set of corporate aims.

Selection criteria could include common conditions; costly interventions, procedures where variations in practice occur and affect patient outcomes, those where there is a high level of interest, those with a changing evidence base, or those areas that commissioners or providers of services identify suitable for attention and development.

The key tasks at this stage are:

- *define goals of the care pathway*—wherever possible, based on evidence of effective practice rather than 'the way we do it round here'
- *team approach*—use a multidisciplinary team approach. Steering groups and working groups should comprise frontline staff, service users, and additional people who have knowledge or expertise in the area
- *developing the team—steering committee*—recognise importance of reaching a common understanding of the function of the group and the parameters within which it will operate. Agree on timescales and communication processes
- *choosing a population, consider as high priority*—high volume, high cost, significant variability in practice, high morbidity/mortality, high public profile, reliance on multidisciplinary team, and demonstrated interest of carers to participate in the process
- *key stakeholders*—determine how to keep stakeholders informed and ensure their concerns are addressed
- *adapt or design?*—two main options are: adapt an existing pathway developed elsewhere or create your own. The NHS Evidence hosts a large database of existing ICPs, which should be consulted before designing your own.[11]

Whatever the 'prime mover' for identifying the need for a care pathway, it is imperative that the identification of the topic is quickly followed by the appointment of the project team. Support for the project should be gained locally—from both commissioner and provider units—which must include the key healthcare team. To obtain engagement at an early stage is essential; the team needs a range of skills as outlined in Box 14.4.

Box 14.4 Project team members and skills
- Management and leadership.
- Clinicians involved in day-to-day delivery of care from a range of professional backgrounds.
- 'Experts' familiar with current evidence base.
- Those providing diagnostic interventions.
- Those providing rehabilitation services.
- Service commissioners.
- Financial modelling skills.
- Patients/carers with experience of receiving care.
- Project management skills.
- Information management and data analysis skills.
- Communication skills.
- Audit skills for ongoing evaluation.
- Support staff.
- Facilitation skills.

Phase 2: review the evidence

The multidisciplinary group needs to undertake a thorough review of the literature, identifying the evidence-based on intervention and caring for the targeted population. The information should be assessed ensuring it meets the requirements for national guidelines and standards where these exist, for example, NICE and NSFs as well as ensuring its relevance to local services.

It is important that some of the team members have skills in undertaking systematic literature reviews. A summary report highlighting key findings and recommendations from the reviewed literature must be drawn up and presented to the rest of the team.

Phase 3: collect data and measure

The importance of accurate data cannot be overemphasised. Data is the keystone to understanding services and improving management of them. Time spent at an early stage collecting accurate, timely, and relevant data will show rewards when analysis and audit of the service improvement is required later.

Measurement is fundamental to any model for service improvement. Having baseline information regarding current clinical practice is an important early step. The team needs to consider current practice rather than assumed practice. It is unlikely that any member of the project team will be fully informed of all the processes and procedures in place. It is important to maintain focus and collect only data directly related to the population under review. This may include economic data—length of stay, cost per case, income, and the number of episodes and contacts—as well as qualitative data from patients and carers.

Gathering data often requires extending the review team to include people experienced in coding and analysis. The complexity is compounded when data gathering extends across organisations and more so if it is needed from other agencies. Sources may also include case note reviews, public health and census statistics, and organisational strategic development plans. Time spent on this exercise is well invested and not a stage that can be missed or compromised.

Measurement—what to measure?

Measurement is an essential part of the process. It is important to develop aims before measuring and to design measures around the aims. Also have clear definitions of measures and measure points, by:

- establishing a reliable baseline
- tracking progress over time
- collecting accurate and complete data
- making results available and feeding back.

Measurement should be used to expedite improvement. It is therefore important to select measures that:

- focus directly on the service being redesigned
- are designed around local and national aims and requirements
- are specific and clearly defined—Specific, Measurable, Achievable, Realistic, and Timed—SMART
- are pragmatic—add value, practical to collect and can be integrated into the daily routine
- are locally agreed and 'owned', not imposed
- incorporate experience from other services where appropriate
- obtain 'buy in' from local stakeholders
- link to improvement work with other initiatives in the health community
- meet requirements of clinical audit and clinical governance.

It is necessary to strike a balance between measures that are feasible to collect and measure the impact of the process change being tested and introduced.

Collecting data

The first stage is to define the starting point or baseline. This will require sufficient time before the improvement work begins. By doing this, it is possible to demonstrate where changes have been beneficial. If no historical data exists, it is important to commence measurement as soon as possible to establish a baseline.

It is a requirement to agree targets that the team wants to achieve and set up a system to monitor progress regularly. The targets must be linked to the aims and objectives agreed. Poor-quality data can invalidate the development process. In order to improve data quality, it is advisable to use it early on in the project—only then will it start to improve.

Use existing data wherever possible. It is important to ensure accuracy, timeliness, relevance, completeness, and consistency for it to be used effectively. It may be necessary to collect the information manually at first. This is the case in many improvement initiatives and gives the chance to learn about the data collection process to ensure that it can be maintained in the longer term.

Sampling is the process of selecting a small representative group in order to draw conclusions about the population or cohort as a whole; this can be a useful technique. A sampling method that minimises bias should be chosen.

When selecting sampling methodology, consider the following factors:
- clinical conditions
- process groups
- age groups
- gender
- time of day/day of week
- sampling technique for example, random, stratified, or a given number.

Once measures have been agreed and data collected, it will be necessary to analyse and present the data to others in the organisation.

A key to successful presentation of information is 'keep it simple'. Charts or diagrams need to be easy to understand. Ideally each element of the presentation should convey one message. Further information on measurement in healthcare is widely available.[11, 13, 14]

Understanding data collection, analysis, and use for AHPs is discussed in detail in the next book of this series, *Managing Money, Measurement and Marketing*.

Phase 4: review current practice including process mapping

There are several methods of implementing change that we have presented and discussed in Chapter 12. The method most widely used in the development of care pathways is process mapping and the model for improvement. This was specifically adapted for use in healthcare by the Institute for Healthcare Improvement in the United States,[15] led by Langley *et al.*[16] The model was subsequently introduced into the NHS by the former Modernisation Agency[17] as one of their tools for service improvement.

The model for improvement was designed to provide a framework for developing, testing, and implementing changes leading to sustainable improvement. It promotes the concept of small-scale study to make bigger sustainable changes. Its framework includes three key questions with a process for testing change ideas using 'Plan, Do, Study, Act' (PDSA) cycles. There are four stages to a PDSA cycle shown in Figure 14.2.

The model has been shown to offer the following benefits:

- it is a simple approach
- it reduces risk by starting small—of particular importance when bringing about changes to clinical systems or care processes
- it can be used to help plan, develop, and implement change

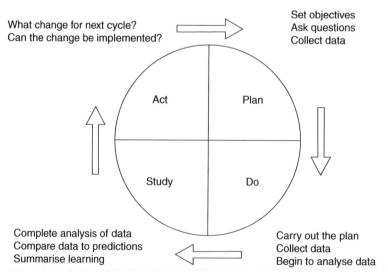

Figure 14.2 Plan do study act cycle—adapted from Langley *et al*[16]

- it supports rapid cycles of improvement
- it can be highly effective
- it supports a 'bottom up' approach to change consistent with systems of continuous improvement
- it can also be used to facilitate large-scale strategic plans.

There are many other successful models of service improvement that may be better suited for ICP development.

Phase 5: identify key indicators

Key indicators are milestones against which to measure progress along a care pathway. They are based on current literature and show where clients should be at specific stages in their care. Indicators must be monitored on a regular basis to ensure that an individual is receiving optimum care. The Canadian Council on Health Services Accreditation defines indicators as:[18]

Measurements, screens, or flags used as a guide to monitor, evaluate, and improve the quality of care, clinical services, support services, and organisational functions that affect client/client outcomes.

Indicators alert the service provider when the activity has reached an acceptable/unacceptable level; for example, waiting times. Indicators may be used as points of reference for evaluation and comparison. They can also be used to examine trends over time. Measuring and reporting of indicators encourages better services, which in turn will improve health outcomes. They are not used for evaluating the performance of individual staff members.

There are three types of indicators: Structure, Process and Outcome shown in Box 14.5.

Box 14.5 Types of key indicators
- **Structure indicators** reflect the environment where the service is provided. These indicators measure the characteristics of care or resources used to provide services to patients. They include the physical facilities, administrative organisation, and qualifications and experience of staff. Environments with good structural properties normally provide quality care and service.
- **Process indicators** reflect the way in which the service is provided. These indicators measure the delivery of care or activities used to provide the service. They include the degree to which the services conform to the standards and expectations of the patient and the provider.
- **Outcome indicators** reflect the achievements of the service. These indicators or measures record the result or end products of care such as levels of mobility and functional ability. They measure the extent to which a desired change, effect, or result was achieved for a patient.

It is important to select the appropriate indicators before the pathway implementation. Monitoring systems need to be set up to collect the range of indicators so that progress can be monitored as a routine rather than as an additional activity.

Phase 6: drafting the care pathway

Algorithm

At this stage, the process of care is analysed and modified to ensure that it is evidence-based and supported by the multidisciplinary team providing care, other service providers, patients/service users, and carers. During this analysis, it is likely that a decision making process will require clarification at some point in the care process. To ensure that the whole team clearly understands the defined process, an algorithm—decision-making tree—should be produced. Algorithms are designed to guide practitioners through the 'if X, then Y' decision making process, which will guide them through the agreed route for intervention to be provided. This in turn ensures that patients are provided with consistent care. Though the algorithm defines the expected pathway for the majority of patients, there is scope for clinical judgment to determine an appropriate deviation from the pathway. An algorithm for Parkinson's disease is shown in Figure 14.3, and for back pain in Figure 14.4.

ICP documentation

Once the care pathway algorithm is agreed, it is possible to proceed to construct a single record of documentation. This includes the multidisciplinary plan and care record that incorporates evidence-based recommendations and indicators—developing a full ICP. All staff involved in the care process will need to contribute to integrating all relevant information from existing documentation. The scale of this task should not be underestimated. The difficulty of developing paperwork that meets the needs of all professional groups and organisations involved can be enormous. Electronic patient records that cross health, education, and social care will, in time, radically change the way that information is recorded, stored, and shared. However, it is necessary to develop paper-based systems in the interim.

Thorough documentation at the outset will avoid the danger of double recording and ensure accurate record-keeping and that pathways meet the organisation's records requirements. The primary documentation form can be used by all members of the care team. It is necessary to ensure that the components of the pathway track the continuum of care—from initial assessment, to care provision and rehabilitation—in both secondary and primary care settings. To enhance and improve the efficiency of the ICP, it is advisable to develop supporting paperwork such as

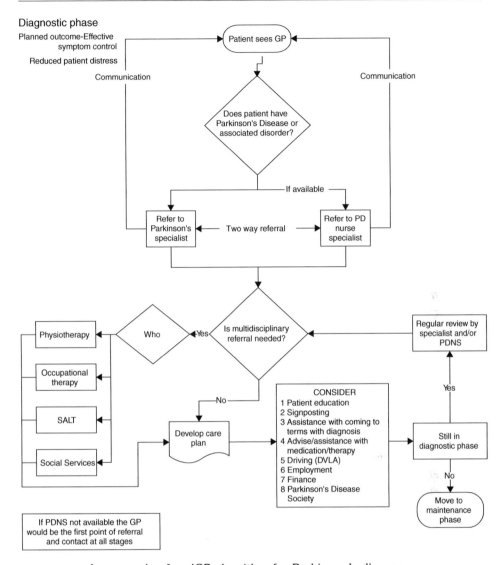

Figure 14.3 An example of an ICP algorithm for Parkinson's disease

standard procedures, patient information, and education materials, as shown in Box 14.6. The documentation may be either 'patient-held' or of the more traditional 'organisation-held' type. The 'patient-held' record should be used by staff and patients to record key information. This might include appointment details, individual goals, medication use diary, strategies, and contingency plans. This record is used to inform the ongoing monitoring and evaluation of the individual's care.

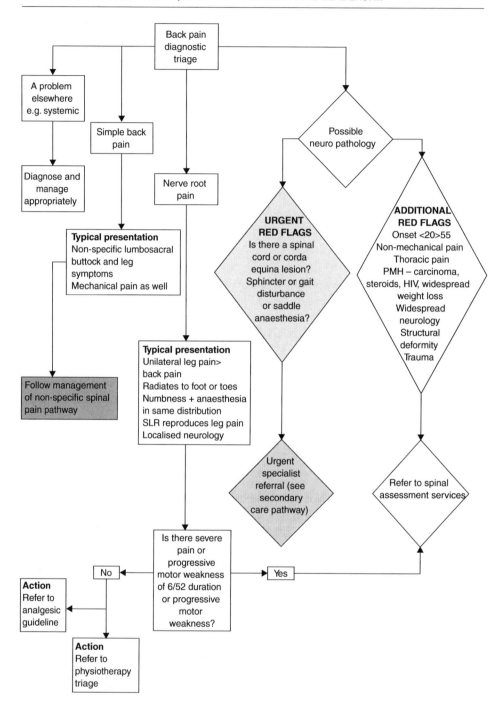

Figure 14.4 An example of an algorithm for back pain

Box 14.6 Items for consideration when developing ICP documentation[19]

A single record of client care.
Standard format.
Simple in design and easy to follow.
Consent.
Abbreviations explained if used.
Include realistic goals, timeframes, and measurable outcomes.
Provide an audit tool.
Wording and content.
Written in plain language.
Include client information.
Highlight roles and accountabilities.
Include signatures of staff.
Dynamics and flexibility.
Incorporate guidelines, protocols, and standards.
Follow a logical sequence, ensuring no duplication.
Easy to complete.
Easy to find relevant information.
Variations recorded together with related actions.

Phase 7: review and revise ICP draft

Once the pathway has been developed, it must be tested before proceeding to full implementation. The final testing enables feedback and suggestions for revisions from other representatives of all relevant disciplines. This input, however, must be considered carefully. If the comments received at this stage deviate from the evidence regarding best practice, it may be necessary to update and inform providers about recommended practices and the research evidence. Testing the revised version of the pathway with a small sample will help identify any further process, design, or system changes required before wider implementation. During this stage, collection of a sample of key indicator data should also be undertaken to check that the care pathway works as intended.

Phase 8: develop user version of care pathway

A user version of the pathway is a useful way to educate and involve patients in the care process. It also provides an opportunity to answer some of the common questions patients are likely to have about their plan of care and various interventions. Use clear language to explain the various steps in the pathway, their projected timing, and, where appropriate, provide key contact names and telephone numbers for further information. User versions are best developed by the users themselves. Examples are shown in Figures 14.5 and 14.6.

The Stroke Care Pathway is designed to be used by the doctors, nurses and therapists who will be taking care of you, the patient, wherever you receive your care (at home, or in either acute or community hospital). This Patient's Version of the Care Pathway is identical, except without a lot of the medical jargon. You should be able to follow what is planned for your care by following the arrows as they lead from one box to the next (see Figure 3.5). The Pathway gives guidance for both clinicians and patients at the main decision points, but it is not intended to provide 'rules' for everything that might happen – that would be impossible, and there may be very good reasons why any particular treatment in your individual case is different. If you are concerned about what is happening or what might happen next you should always try to discuss this with your doctor, nurse or therapist – they will want to know what is worrying you.

As the process of stroke care develops this care pathway will be updated. For comments and feedback contact the xxxx

Some common questions people ask about stroke and Transient Ischaemic Attack (TIA)

What is a stroke?

A stroke is an illness in which part of the brain is suddenly severely damaged or destroyed. This causes a loss of function of the affected part of the brain. It usually causes weakness, paralysis of the arm and leg on either the left or right side of the body, twisting of the face, and in some cases other effects which may include loss of balance, disturbance of vision, disturbance of speech, loss of control of the bladder and bowels, and difficulty in swallowing. In very severe cases, there is a loss of consciousness or confusion of thought. The damage in the brain is caused by a blood clot or a haemorrhage.

What is a transient ischaemic attack ('TIA')?

A transient ischaemic attack or TIA is very like a stroke except that it passes quickly; the symptoms of weakness of one side of the body, tingling and twisting of the mouth or loss of speech or disturbance of vision last only for a few minutes or hours and then disappear. TIAs occur because, for a short time, not enough blood reaches part of the brain. They can be treated and anyone who experiences a TIA should see their doctor.

What is the risk of another stroke?

Life is a risky business, and if we thought about risk the whole time we would never cross the road or go up in an aeroplane. While there is no good reason to assume that one stroke will inevitably be followed by another, the condition that caused the first – such as high blood pressure – will need treating to reduce the chances of the same condition causing another stroke. After an ischaemic stroke (see box, top right), you will be prescribed aspirin to reduce the risk of another stroke.

It is best to try to train oneself to treat the fear of another stroke in the same way as you treat the danger of a crash when you buy an air ticket - it could happen, yes, but it probably won't.

Why should I have a six-month check-up?

It is strongly recommended that six months after your stroke, wherever you are living by then, you go back to your doctor or nurse at the surgery or health centre for a check-up. The doctor or nurse will want to check on your recovery from the stroke; they will want to check your medication and to see that everything is being done to reduce your risk of another stroke; and to see whether there is any need for more therapy for you.

What causes a stroke?

Most strokes occur in the second half of life and are caused by damage to the blood vessels – and sometimes to the heart – which has been building up slowly for many years. Most strokes happen when a blood clot forms in a damaged vessel and blocks the flow of blood to part of the brain (an *ischaemic* stroke), but some happen when a damaged blood vessel in the brain bursts and blood pours from it into the brain itself (a *haemorrhagic* stroke).

In at least half of all strokes the reason why the blood vessels become damaged in the first place is because they have been exposed to high blood pressure. If in addition the patient smokes, drinks heavily, is over-weight, takes too much salt in their diet, or has heart disease or diabetes the risk of stroke is increased. A number of other factors are suspected, but there is no single cause of stroke, and some strokes even happen without a cause ever being found.

Anyone can suffer a stroke at any time, although the risks can be substantially reduced by a healthy life style, including the avoidance of smoking, and especially by having your blood pressure checked and, if it is too high, ensuring that it is kept under control by treatment.

Why should I go to a Stroke Unit instead of my local hospital?

Research work over the last thirty years shows that people with stroke stand a better chance of surviving if they are cared for on a Stroke Unit. They also stand a better chance of recovering well enough to return home after the stroke. Because of this, the NHS runs a specialist Stroke Unit at the local hospital for the 'acute' period of care (generally the first week), so almost all people with stroke would go there first. After that, care is provided in the Stroke Rehabilitation Unit, or in your local community hospital. There, treatment and rehabilitation will continue, and if all goes well, plans can be made for your return home. If you need it, therapy can continue after you get home with therapists who can see you either as an out patient or in the community.

How can I get more information?

You should find that most of your questions about stroke and TIA can be answered by the health staff who are looking after you. Information can also be obtained from the Stroke Association, an independent national charity for people after a stroke and their carers, which runs telephone helplines and provides publications and welfare grants, and has affiliated local stroke clubs. The national website is www.stroke.org.uk. This Patient Version of the Care Pathway has been prepared with the help of local stroke patients and the Stroke Association.

Figure 14.5 An example of patient produced information

Phase 9: launching care pathways

The launch of an ICP will have a significant bearing on its success. A poorly launched care pathway will not be well used or adhered to and therefore have limited impact on patient care. It is essential to plan the launch as part of the project planning; this is one of the most essential milestones and is necessary to engage a much wider

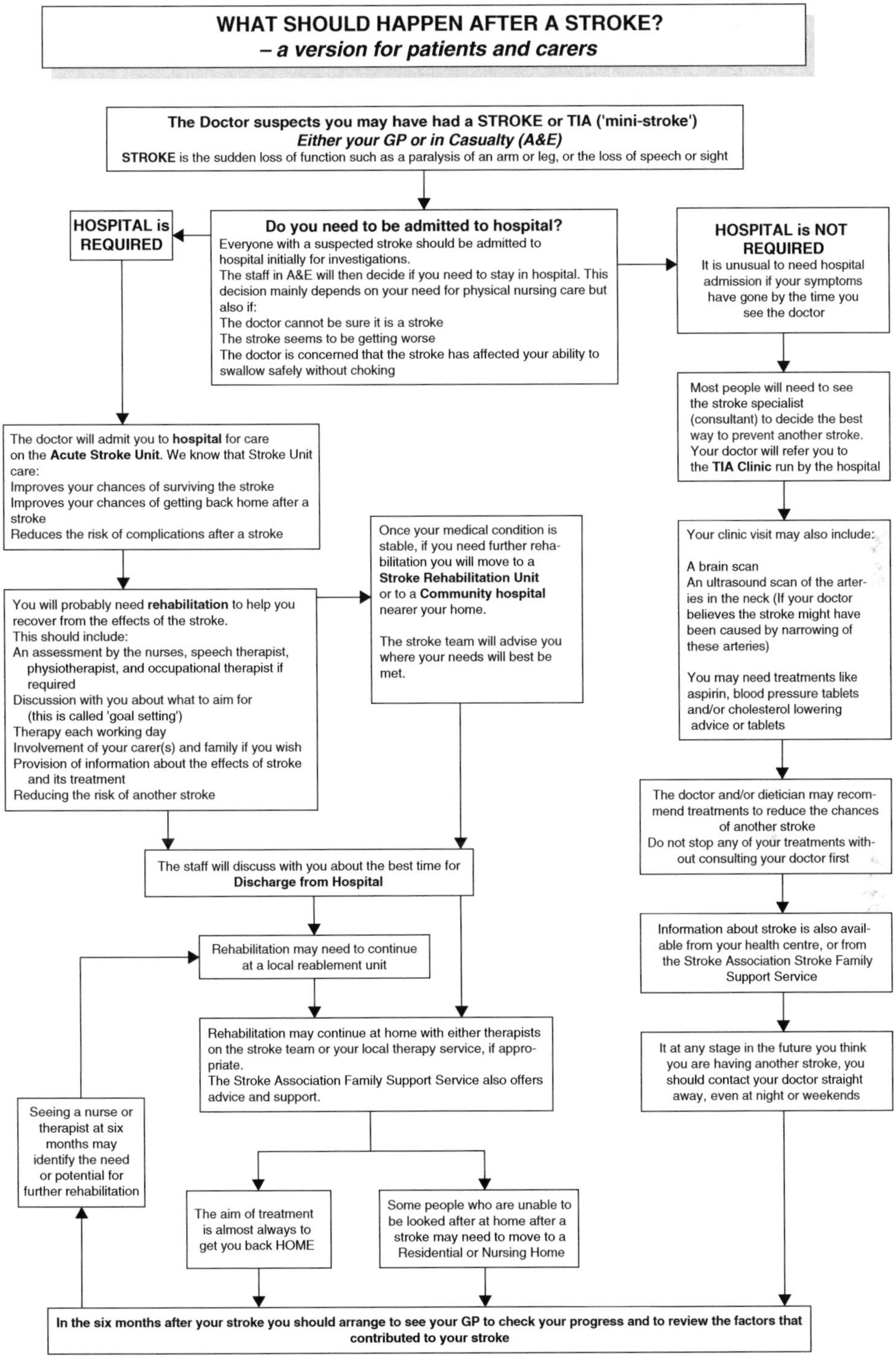

WHAT SHOULD HAPPEN AFTER A STROKE?
– a version for patients and carers

The Doctor suspects you may have had a STROKE or TIA ('mini-stroke')
Either your GP or in Casualty (A&E)
STROKE is the sudden loss of function such as a paralysis of an arm or leg, or the loss of speech or sight

HOSPITAL is REQUIRED

Do you need to be admitted to hospital?
Everyone with a suspected stroke should be admitted to hospital initially for investigations.
The staff in A&E will then decide if you need to stay in hospital. This decision mainly depends on your need for physical nursing care but also if:
The doctor cannot be sure it is a stroke
The stroke seems to be getting worse
The doctor is concerned that the stroke has affected your ability to swallow safely without choking

HOSPITAL is NOT REQUIRED
It is unusual to need hospital admission if your symptoms have gone by the time you see the doctor

Most people will need to see the stroke specialist (consultant) to decide the best way to prevent another stroke. Your doctor will refer you to the **TIA Clinic** run by the hospital

The doctor will admit you to **hospital** for care on the **Acute Stroke Unit**. We know that Stroke Unit care:
Improves your chances of surviving the stroke
Improves your chances of getting back home after a stroke
Reduces the risk of complications after a stroke

Once your medical condition is stable, if you need further rehabilitation you will move to a **Stroke Rehabilitation Unit** or to a **Community hospital** nearer your home.

The stroke team will advise you where your needs will best be met.

Your clinic visit may also include:

A brain scan
An ultrasound scan of the arteries in the neck (If your doctor believes the stroke might have been caused by narrowing of these arteries)

You may need treatments like aspirin, blood pressure tablets and/or cholesterol lowering advice or tablets

You will probably need **rehabilitation** to help you recover from the effects of the stroke.
This should include:
An assessment by the nurses, speech therapist, physiotherapist, and occupational therapist if required
Discussion with you about what to aim for (this is called 'goal setting')
Therapy each working day
Involvement of your carer(s) and family if you wish
Provision of information about the effects of stroke and its treatment
Reducing the risk of another stroke

The doctor and/or dietician may recommend treatments to reduce the chances of another stroke
Do not stop any of your treatments without consulting your doctor first

The staff will discuss with you about the best time for **Discharge from Hospital**

Information about stroke is also available from your health centre, or from the Stroke Association Stroke Family Support Service

Rehabilitation may need to continue at a local reablement unit

Rehabilitation may continue at home with either therapists on the stroke team or your local therapy service, if appropriate.
The Stroke Association Family Support Service also offers advice and support.

It at any stage in the future you think you are having another stroke, you should contact your doctor straight away, even at night or weekends

Seeing a nurse or therapist at six months may identify the need or potential for further rehabilitation

The aim of treatment is almost always to get you back HOME

Some people who are unable to be looked after at home after a stroke may need to move to a Residential or Nursing Home

In the six months after your stroke you should arrange to see your GP to check your progress and to review the factors that contributed to your stroke

Figure 14.6 Patient version of care pathway

audience than during the developmental stages. The pathway will have a much greater impact if time is spent ensuring that those people who will use it in their day-to-day work understand the benefits and do not see it as 'just another pathway'. A robust launch strategy will improve the chances of successful implementation.

The strategy should identify the key stages of implementation and actions. The strategy should offer a checklist of tasks that are shared among the implementation group.

- **Communication:** It is vital that people who will be asked to work in a different way following the introduction of the pathway are supported. Many good pathways falter due to the concerns of staff, who may regard the pathway as an imposition threatening their clinical freedom. The pathway may require staff to work with some agencies or services for the first time. It is important to the implementation to invest time in discussing and understanding the issues around professional regulation and accountability as well as exploring areas of commonality. Provide time in the implementation strategy to explore fully the potential benefits of the care pathway with the people who will be asked to implement it and the service users who will experience it. A key 'selling' point is the underlying objective to improve the quality of care that is evidence-based.

- **Awareness:** All staff using the pathway require information about the practical aspects of implementation. In addition, the executive teams need to be made aware of the care pathway and its launch in order to ensure support at board level. All relevant staff should have access to awareness sessions or briefings covering the principles of the pathway; the practicalities of how to work within it and how to make the most of it.

  It is often difficult to get everyone together at the same time to provide a formal awareness session. Multiple methods for briefing should be considered. These may include, for example:

  - a formal launch at an event solely planned to begin the use of the new pathway. This is a good way to get a large group of staff together, but it will be impossible to gather everyone who need to be aware of the ICP
  - 'road shows' where a few members of the steering group go to meet key staff at, for example, departmental meetings, practice meetings, or voluntary organisations meetings
  - putting the care pathway onto a Web page
  - e-mailing the pathway to key contacts
  - writing the pathway onto a CD
  - making paper copies available and sending to named individuals.

- **Timing:** Ensure that the launch of the ICP doesn't clash with other events that may detract from the impact of the launch.

- **Resources:** ICP development requires significant resource input, especially in staff time. The launch itself will also need to be funded; do not underestimate the administration time required. It is important to invite a wide range of people, for example, pathway users, carers, commissioners, the multidisciplinary team, voluntary sector, and communications leads. Record the names of all those who attend the launch sessions, as gaps in representation can subsequently be followed up. There may be costs for room hire, refreshments, printing, copying, and so on. Sponsorship can be mutually advantageous, but will depend on local circumstances and procedures.

Documentation

An integral part of all care pathways is thorough documentation. However, some pathways do not incorporate specifically designed multidisciplinary record-keeping system, but many do. The principles of good quality documentation and record-keeping apply equally to ICPs as they do to traditional recording systems. Middleton and Roberts[19] report that there is consensus regarding ICP documentation, which should be:

- sequential, specifying timing and indicators how to move along the pathway
- written in plain language, avoiding abbreviations where possible.

They further suggest that there are two reasons why new documentation is likely to take more time to complete, neither of which is likely to continue in the long term.

- Any new system requires familiarisation time. The act of having to turn pages over to find where to write a particular piece of information rather than writing it down on the next piece of blank paper will be more time consuming until staff are able to turn to the required place automatically.
- ICPs may require some staff to write more than they did before, particularly in situations where previous documentation was not well completed and where routine notes about patients' progress were not kept to an adequate standard.

ICP documentation must meet the requirements of the legal care record, which can be challenging, particularly when some care may be provided away from where the notes are held. For this reason, some services implement ICPs without integrating record-keeping systems. However, it is recommended that wherever possible, a single record of care should be implemented. The electronic patient record will in time facilitate the use of one clinical record for all staff.

Decreasing the administrative burden for health and social care staff is a welcome by-product of a well-structured ICP. Documentation is concerned with anticipating the 'routine' of care, thereby guiding the practitioner to follow what is anticipated. Although the content of individual ICPs differs, there are benefits to be gained by keeping to a standardised format. This might include:

- front page for patient details such as name and demographic information
- consent
- clinical assessment—including risk assessment
- care plan and patient management notes—which may be colour-coded for ease of navigation
- discharge planning
- variations from the expected pathway.

Comprehensive advice on the design of care pathway documentation is provided by de Luc.[20]

Phase 10: monitor indicators—review and amend

It is important to establish a system for monitoring indicators in the care pathway. The method used depends on the stage of the pathway development and processes or outcomes being monitored.

- Implementation evaluation: In the initial stages of implementation, it may be necessary to frequently monitor several of the intended pathway indicators to identify problems in the pathway itself. Once the pathway is established and implementation issues have been resolved, it can then be evaluated and revised to reflect new evidence and 'best' practices.
- Individual patient progress: These indicators relate to individual patients' progress along the pathway. Variations in the expected course at any stage will have implications for subsequent steps in the care process.
- Patient group outcome: These indicators relate to the entire group for which the pathway has been developed. These outcomes help identify 'bottlenecks' and constraints facilitating quality of care reporting, for example, waiting times and length of stay.

EVALUATION OF CARE PATHWAYS

Analysis and review are essential processes in the evaluation of the effectiveness of care pathways. This also contributes to the cycle of continuous improvement and ensures that care and interventions are based on current evidence of effective practice.

Not only do indicators need monitoring, but the pathway itself needs maintaining. Pathways will continually evolve. If the care pathway is going to be used to promote continuous service improvement, resources including staff need to be assigned to this work.

To maintain momentum, de Luc[20] suggests elements that need to be put in place.

Box 14.7 Checklist for pathway maintenance
- Nominate a person to lead the maintenance process.
- Ensure arrangements in place for production of revised pathway and updating.
- Where a paper recording system is used, ensure ongoing supplies.
- Nominate a care pathway trainer.
- Put in place a training programme for new staff and updates for existing staff.
- Ensure staff are monitored for accuracy and timeliness of completing pathway.
- Set up an audit plan.
- Set dates for audit meetings for the multidisciplinary team.
- Agree to a review date for the care pathway content, including user views.

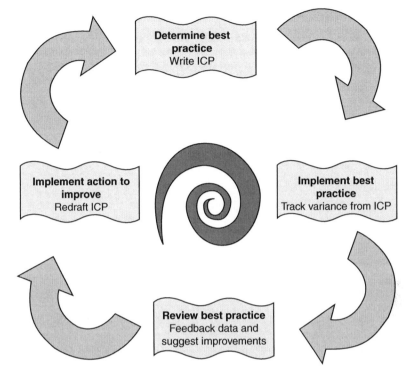

Figure 14.7 A care pathway continuous cycle of improvement

THE PURPOSE OF ANALYSIS AND REVIEW

Before commencing the process, it is necessary to identify several key indicators, including:

- has the implementation of this pathway improved patient care?
- has it provided at least the same level of care at no more cost than previously?
- are there any changes that can be made which will improve its effectiveness?

It is also important to identify learning points arising during the course of a pathway, particularly those issues around partnership and collaborative working.

Middleton and Roberts[19] identify a number of possible areas to examine during a care pathway review:

- changes in documentation, that is, accuracy, completeness, and amount of time required to complete
- changes in care provision or process of care, for example, introduction of guidelines, increased consistency, length of stay, number of contacts, shortening time delays, reducing number of contacts, and changes in who provides care
- changes in patient and staff satisfaction
- changes in outcomes of care.

HOW TO USE CARE PATHWAYS

Once a care pathway has been developed, all staff are expected to implement it. This will require them to:
- follow the care pathway for every patient within the specified care group
- use appropriate documentation and record interventions and pathway progress
- justify any deviation from the pathway and indicate the reasons for variation
- take appropriate action when progress deviates from that anticipated in the pathway
- ensure patients and carers understand the pathway and its application to them.

BENEFITS AND BARRIERS

Some of the possible benefits and barriers to successful implementation of care pathways are listed in Box 14.8. If the benefits do not outweigh the barriers, then it may indicate that the wrong clinical area is being addressed. There has been a lot of evaluation of ICPs, with more than 4000 international references to the use of them and more than 45 different care group or diagnosis related pathways in use in the UK.[3] In addition to the benefits listed, there are reported additional benefits of improved patient outcomes, quality of life and reduced complications,[21] reduced length of stay in hospital, increased patient satisfaction,[19] reduction of cost of care,[22] improved inter-disciplinary communication, and reduction of time taken by staff to complete paperwork. The latter point is worthy of note; as many clinicians consider at the outset, that note keeping time will be increased. However, due to the multi-disciplinary nature of the care pathway, duplication of assessment is significantly reduced, resulting in overall less time required for record-keeping.

Box 14.8 Benefits and barriers to care pathway implementation

Key benefits
1 Facilitate the introduction of protocols based on evidence.
2 Promote more patient-centred care—improving patient involvement.
3 Facilitate interdisciplinary working.
4 Improve care planning and monitoring.
5 Improve multidisciplinary audit.
6 Enable changing evidence base to be quickly incorporated into practice.
7 Identified areas for individual clinician improvement.
8 Identified areas for whole service improvement.
9 Make better use of resources.
10 Improved service attracts more business.
11 Improved record-keeping.
12 Improved clinical governance.
13 Provides equity of access and care.
14 Consistency and simplicity of commissioning.
15 Quality-assured services.

Possible barriers

1 Appear prescriptive.
2 Reduce clinical freedom.
3 Be a resistance to change.
4 Appear to be a cost saving initiative rather than one of quality improvement.
5 Be difficult to obtain staff engagement and 'ownership'.
6 Unrealistic time frame.
7 Obstructive interpersonal politics.
8 Fail to be adopted if communication is poor.
9 Require significant service redesign.
10 Require investment of resources.
11 Lack leadership and project management skills.
12 Not gain commissioner support.
13 Conflicting organisational priorities.

The barriers are not insurmountable. However, it is essential to recognise the importance of some of these, because if they are not addressed, they may impede progress or prevent completion of the pathway. Clinician resistance can be a major barrier to pathway development and implementation. Recognising that the change process gives rise to question the way that care is currently provided—suggesting that current practice is not optimal—is an important factor. Skilful leadership is necessary to gain support from those staff keen to make the required changes, without alienating those who are slower to adapt and engage. Initially, it is better to work with a small group of enthusiasts, rather than trying to persuade the wider team that the change programme is of value. One-to-one work with 'resistant' clinicians will give opportunity to find common ground and is a tactic worth exploring.

If, for example, significant service redesign is required to implement the new pathway and the timing is not right to embark on a major project, it might be better to delay implementation rather than fail. Therefore, awareness of the possible barriers aids selection of the right care pathway to develop. Undoubtedly it is better to do this at the beginning of the process rather than at the end.

CONCLUSION

There is strong evidence that the experience of health professionals both in the UK and United States points to benefits of using care pathways.[23] For pathways to be successfully adopted, they must be accurately completed and audited. Any deficiencies uncovered need to be remedied during the review stage. This rigor ensures that pathways remain live processes fulfilling the purpose of providing evidence-based care for patients.

Arguably the best examples of care pathways tend to have several things in common; they frequently:

- examine the best evidence; locally, nationally, and internationally
- use local knowledge, experience, and expertise
- involve service users in the design and evaluation processes
- involve a number of different disciplines in a team decision, creating 'ownership'
- use continuous improvement models
- ensure teams have information for feedback on a regular basis
- review and amend the pathway in light of audit results or changing evidence-base and feedback.

There is a wealth of information available to assist, inform, and guide pathway developers.[1, 8, 10, 14, 15, 17, 18, 24, 25, 26, 27, 28, 29] There are, however, criticisms of ICPs, and it is recognised that there is a need to develop more evidence about their effectiveness. McDonald *et al*[22] assert that:

ICPs are helpful in achieving consensus on the consistency and continuity of care and can improve the documentation of evidence-based and patient focused care. The standard of ICPs is variable and, although their use is now widespread, they have not been meaningfully evaluated. Failures to identify improvements in care following the introduction of an ICP have been linked to their implementation and variability in content quality. Although there are a large number of integrated care pathways listed on NHS Evidence, no 'kite mark' has been used to assure a sound clinical, managerial, ethical, and legal footing for them, although Map of Medicine[27] has been widely adopted as the best source of up-to-date evidence-based pathways providing more than 400 maps available internationally, though locally modifiable.

Care pathways are reported to result in the provision of better quality care and almost always manage to do this at lower cost.[1] Cost containment itself may be a benefit, but equitable better quality care should remain the key objective. AHPs are an essential staff group in the development of care pathways, and we advise AHPs to embrace the concept of care pathways, contributing their management, leadership, and clinical expertise by participating fully in the design and implementation process.

REFERENCES

1. Roy S. Foreword. In: De Luc K, editor. *Developing Care Pathways—the handbook.* Oxford: Radcliffe Medical Press; 2001.
2. www.jr2.ox.ac.uk/bandolier/Extraforbando/Forum2.pdf; 2003.
3. Campbell H, Hotchkiss R, Porteous M. Integrated care pathways. www.the-npa.org.uk.
4. European Pathway Association. Slovenia Board Meeting; December 2005. www.e-p-a.org/index2.html.
5. Overill S. A practical guide to care pathways. *Int J Integr Care.* 1998; 2: 93–8.
6. www.evidence-based-medicine.co.uk/.
7. Wilson J. *An Introduction to Multi-Disciplinary Pathways of Care.* Newcastle: Northern Regional Health Authority; 1992.

8. www.the-npa.org.uk.
9. Coffey R, Richards J, Remmert C, *et al.* An introduction to critical paths. *Qual Manag Health Care.* 1992; **1**: 45–54.
10. Kitchiner D, Davidson C, Bundred P. Integrated care pathways; effective tools for continuous evaluation of clinical practice. *J Eval Clin Prac.* 1996; **2**(1): 65–9.
11. www.library.nhs.uk/default.aspx.
12. Audit Commission. *Governing Partnerships. Bridging the Accountability Gap.* London: HMSO; 2005.
13. Campbell H. Integrated care pathways increase use of guideline. www.bmj.bmjjournals.com/cgi/content/full/317/7151/147/b.
14. www.venturetc.com/eicps.asp.
15. The Institute for Healthcare Improvement, USA. www.ihi.org.
16. Langley G, Nolan K, Nolan T, *et al. The Improvement Guide: a practical approach to enhancing organisational performance.* San Francisco: Jossey-Bass Publishers; 1996.
17. NHS Institute for Innovation and Improvement. www.institute.nhs.uk/.
18. www.cchsa.ca/upload/files/pdf/ISQua/Introduction.pdf.
19. Middleton S, Roberts A. *Integrated Care Pathways: a practical approach to implementation.* London: Butterworth-Heinemann; 2000.
20. De Luc K. *Developing Care Pathways—the tool kit.* Oxford: Radcliffe Medical Press; 2001.
21. www.library.nhs.uk/pathways.
22. McDonald P, Whittle C, Dunn L, *et al.* Shortfalls in integrated care pathways: part 1: what don't they contain? *J Integ Care Pathways.* 2006; **10**(1): 17–22.
23. Mosher C, Cronk P, Kidd A, *et al.* Upgrading practice with critical pathways. *Am J Nurs* 1992; **1**: 41–4.
24. The National Assembly of Wales. *An introduction to Clinical Pathways, Putting Patients First.* Cardiff: HMSO; 1999.
25. Stead L, Arthur C, Cleary A. Do multi-disciplinary pathways of care affect patient satisfaction? *Health Care Risk Report.* 1995; **Nov**: 13–5.
26. Trubo R. If this is cookbook medicine, you may like it. *Medical Economics* 1993; **69**: 69–82.
27. www.mapofmedicine.com.
28. Currie L, Harvey G. *The Origins and Use of Care Pathways in the USA, Australia, and the United Kingdom.* Report 15. Oxford: Royal College of Nursing Institute; 1998.
29. The Centre for Change and Innovation. www.cci.scot.nhs.uk.

FURTHER READING

• Zander K. Integrated Care Pathways: eleven international trends. *J Integ Care Pathways.* 2002; **6**:101–7.
• Harkleroad A, Schirf D, Volpe J, *et al.* Critical pathway development: An integrative literature review. *Am J Occup Ther.* 2000; **54**(2): 148–54.
Chartered Society of Physiotherapy. *International Journal of Care Pathways*, Available at : http://ijcp.rsmjournals.com/.
• Trowbridge R, Weingarten S. *Making Health Care Safer, A Critical Analysis of Patient Safety Practices.* Chapter 52: Critical Pathways. Agency for Healthcare Research and Quality, 2001.
• Van Herck P, Vanhaecht K, Sermeus W. Effects of clinical pathways: do they work? *J Integ Care Pathways* 2004; **8**: 95–105.

CHAPTER 15

Top tips for report writing

Fiona Jenkins and Robert Jones

Writing successfully takes practice and is a skill in itself. The following list outlines some tips we have found helpful.

Box 15.1 Checklist for report writing

- The faster and easier your audience receives your key messages, the more successful your report will be.
- Know your audience—beware of jargon and do not over estimate or underestimate their technical understanding of the topic.
- Signpost your document to facilitate reading, as a good content page and headings are essential—do not assume the audience will be as keen to read it as you were to write it.
- Give attention to the title page; make it stand out.
- Write a short summary—one or two sentences that give the condensed version of your whole document; this helps you focus.
- Make sure you ask the reader for the action you are wanting—not just a passive essay.
- Give the reader a date by which action is required.
- Write for the reader who 'scans' and make sure headings convey the key points.
- Do not make it too long! It may never get read.
- Make sure you explain the benefits of your request, make good use of the appendices.
- Avoid telling the readers what they already know.
- Avoid negative text—turn it around to be positive with a solution to the problem.

- Keep sentences short. Use bullets effectively, but not repeatedly, and never more than six bullets.
- Figures and tables—number them and use strong headings to convey key messages.
- Avoid pointless words—like 'basically', 'actually', and 'undoubtedly'. They add nothing to the message and often can be removed without changing the meaning or the tone. You will find sentences survive, succeed, and may even flourish without them.
- Focus the conclusion and recommendations section—have you drawn together all the main ideas without adding in new information?
- Do not forget references and acknowledgements and use a consistent style.
- Write a draft report and get someone to read it and give you honest feedback.

CHAPTER 16

Top tips for report presentation

Robert Jones and Fiona Jenkins

Box 16.1 Checklist for report presentation

Skill 1—be sure of your objectives
- Have an objective in mind for your presentation and think about the objectives of your audience.
- Make sure you know about the group, who they are and what their levels of knowledge/experience is, why the presentation is taking place, what the audience is hoping to gain from it.
- Decide what style of presentation is appropriate.

Skill 2—be prepared
- Preparation is key to success in any presentation.
- Allow plenty of time for preparation.
- Know who the audience are.
- Speak to the event organisers before the event.
- Know the roles of people in the audience in respect of influence, authority, and decision-making.
- Know why individuals are at the presentation.
- What do you know about the 'agendas' of those attending—why are they there?
- Who supports you, and who is potentially against you?
- What objections can you expect and what arguments or strategies have you got to rebut them?
- If more than one of you is involved in making the presentation, who will lead on which areas and why?

Presentation checklist:
- phones off
- someone on the door to welcome
- is there a fire alarm test due!
- room layout and seating/tables
- no barriers—take control of the space
- break times if a long presentation
- lighting arrangements
- timing
- stand, lectern where appropriate
- projector table positioning
- test all audio media equipment
- have spare handouts where appropriate
- rehearse if you can

Skill 3—have structure
- Keep it simple and straightforward
- Strategies for eliciting:
- Why?
  - Universal truths
  - Stories and metaphors
  - Rhetorical questions
  - Ask the audience
  - Discussions
  - Recap
- What?
  - What are the key points to be covered?
  - What are the main elements of each point?
  - What is the right level of detail for this audience?
  - If selling (or an idea) what are the benefits of what you are proposing/ selling?
  - Focus on tangible results and softer intangible benefits.
  - Repeat and emphasise key points.
- How will it work?
  - Examples.
  - Using demonstrations, models, graphs, and figures.
  - Getting them to do it—role play where appropriate.
  - Doing an exercise, apply to real situations with examples.
  - Getting them to talk about how they could use this—with others in the audience.
  - Drawing, writing, and brainstorming.

- Questions.
  - Always summarise the benefits.
  - Focus on the core benefits.
  - Call to action.
  - Recommend future actions and agree on next steps where appropriate.

Skill 4—take notes with you
- Never rely on the PowerPoint—it may not work!
- Use brief notes of salient points.
- Use mind mapping for planning presentations.

Skill 5—use engaging language
- Do not be long-winded.
- Use straightforward (not overcomplicated) words.
- Create audience involvement.
- Use signposts—let people know what's coming.
- Be positive.
- Talk about benefits.
- Avoid vague, wishy-washy words.
- Avoid useless phrases.
- Avoid being overly technical or complex.

Skill 6—use presentation aids appropriately
- No one likes 'death by PowerPoint'.
- PowerPoint should only aid, illustrate, and serve to spice up; it should never be used as an *aide-mémoire*.
- Use a variety of presentation slides, not just words.
- Handouts.
  - Must be 'branded' and must be clear they are presentation material.
  - Should leave room for note taking.
  - Should expand on the bullet points on the screen, not just reiterate them.
  - Can be used actively during the presentation: 'now, what I want you to do is ....
  - Must be something they will want to keep.

Skill 7—engage your audience
- Speak to some people early on as they arrive if you can.
- Smile, make eye contact.
- Learn some names if you have chance.
- Bring people in—walk around, own the territory.
- Use 'fizzy' exercises, ask questions, divide into groups, ask for volunteers, vote on something, give something away, or play a game.
- Use 'yes' sets.

- Ask questions.
- Look for energisers.
- Watch your body language: symmetrical, upright, palms down, hands moving down and outward from chest level, open, asymmetrical, leaning forward.
- Never turn your back to the audience to read from the screen!
- Go there first, whenever possible go to the presentation room first, claim the area, and make it your own.

Skill 8—take questions and deal with challenges
- Questions are a sign your audience is 'still there' and interested.
- Ask questions yourself.
- Listen and demonstrate that you are listening through your body language.
- Ask individuals to repeat or elaborate.
- Ask others their opinions.
- Be honest.
- Prepare answers to likely questions.

Skill 9—get the edge
- Avoid monotonous pitch.
- Consider the emotion behind key messages examples and sentences.
- Be slow to drive home key points and benefits.
- Use pauses for emphasis.
- Seek feedback and listen to feedback non-judgmentally.
- Enjoy! If you enjoy the presentation, your audience probably will, too.

CHAPTER 17

Templates

Robert Jones and Fiona Jenkins

Template17.1 AHP Services Clinical Governance
Quarterly Report Template
Reporting Period: Year: 20....... Quarter: ....
Please note that all tables in the templates can have extra rows inserted according to local need

SECTION 1 – ROLLING LOG AND RISK REGISTER

Rolling Log

Date of Meeting	Action Point/Issue	Outstanding Issue	Resolution Plan	Lead	Target Date	Resolution Plan Implemented	Further Action Necessary?	Assurance	Score

Risk Register

ID No	Title of Risk	Opened	Site	Description	Risk level (initial)	Rating (current)	Rating (initial)	Closed date

SECTION 2 – NICE GUIDELINES (Source Nice Guidance Report)

All NICE guidance for AHPs will be reviewed for compliance.

Title	Action/Date

SECTION 3 – INFECTION CONTROL –

Infection Control Issue	Action Required/Date

SECTION 4 – SERIOUS UNTOWARD INCIDENTS (SUIs)

SUI ID NUMBER	DATE OF INCIDENT	REPORT DUE DATE	DIRECTORATE	SPECIALITY	CATEGORY	INCIDENT UPDATE/ PROGRESS	LESSONS LEARNT

SECTION 5 – RISK FEEDBACK

Clinical Incidents

Location 1	Month 1	Month 2	Month 3	Total	Total same period previous Year.....
Number of reported incidents					
Total Number of on-going incidents as at Month/Year					

Location 2	Month 1	Month 2	Month 3	Total	Total same period previous Year ......
Number of reported incidents					
Total Number of on-going incidents as at Month/Year					

Top 10 Incidents Year: 20.......... Quarter ....

Category	Location	Number

SECTION 6 - NPSA - NATIONAL PATIENT SAFETY ALERT BULLETINS (SAB's)

National Patient Safety Alerts
Central Alerting System (CAS) Safety Alerts
Received from the Medicine and Healthcare Regulatory Authority (MHRA)

Title of Safety Alert	Action Required/Date

SECTION 7 - COMPLAINTS AND PATIENT'S ADVISORY LIAISON SERVICE OR EQUIVALENT
(Source – Complaints/PALs Office and Local Records)

Complaints

Ref	Site	Specialty (Subjects)	Incident date	First received	Closed	Reopened	Description	Outcome

PALS Contacts

New PALS contacts received in the quarter: Location 1 =   Location 2 =

New PALS contacts received this quarter by subject:

Subject	Location 1	Location 2
Grand Total		

Please note that an enquiry or complaint may relate to more than one subject

New PALS concerns received this quarter by specialty:

Specialty	Location 1	Location 2
Grand Total		

Please note that an enquiry or complaint may relate to more than one specialty

Number of Plaudits Received

Quarter ...., Year.........	Specialty 1	Specialty 2	Specialty 3
Month 1			
Month 2			
Month 3			
Total			

SECTION 8 – PATIENT INFORMATION – REVIEWED THIS QUARTER

Title of Information	Action/Date

SECTION 9 – NATIONAL AUDITS AND REPORTS

Title of Audit/Report	Action/date

SECTION 10 – LOCAL AUDITS

The following audits were completed during the quarter:

Audit No.	Lead	Site	Title	Completion date	Recommendations/ Actions	Actions implemented?

The following audits were started or ongoing during the quarter:

Audit No.	Lead	Site	Title	Status as at..........	Anticipated completion date

SECTION 11 – CLAIMS (Source of Information Legal Department)

Medical negligence claims –
Liability claims –

SECTION 12 –

H&S Risk Assessments Undertaken

	Month 1	Month 2	Month 3
New Risk Assessments			
Risk Assessment due for review			

Details of risk assessments due for review

Ref No	Site	Department	Hazard	Risk	Date of Risk Assessment	Review Due

Policies Overdue and Reviewed

Database no.	Document Title	Responsible Clinician/author	Review due date	Next review date	Comments

Attendance at risk meetings

Date scheduled	Site	Held yes/no	Attendance	Manager/H&S present?

SECTION 13 – COMMENTS

Template 17.2 AHP Human Resources Performance Report Therapy Services Directorate year....
Workforce

Appraisal								
		Appraisal Compliance (%)						
		Red < 70%, Amber 70% – 85%, Green > 85%						
Organisation %	**Directorate**	**Dietetics**	**O.T**	**Orthotics**	**Physio**	**Podiatry**	**SLT**	**Comments**
May								
June								
July								
Aug								
Sept								
Oct								
Nov								
Dec								
Jan								
Feb								
March								
April								

Mandatory Training

Red < 80%, Amber 80% – 90%, Green > 90%

Organisation	Induction	Fire	Manual Handling	Infection Control
Apr				
May				
June				
July				
Aug				
Sept				
Oct				
Nov				
Dec				
Jan				
Feb				
March				

Red < 80%, Amber 80% – 90%, Green > 90%

Therapies	Induction	Fire	Manual Handling	Infection Control
Apr				
May				
June				
July				
Aug				
Sept				
Oct				
Nov				
Dec				
Jan				
Feb				
March				

O.T	Induction	Fire	Manual Handling	Infection Control
Apr				
May				
June				
July				
Aug				
Sept				
Oct				
Nov				
Dec				
Jan				
Feb				
March				

Dietetics	Induction	Fire	Manual Handling	Infection Control
Apr				
May				
June				
July				
Aug				
Sept				
Oct				
Nov				
Dec				
Jan				
Feb				
March				

Physio	Induction	Fire	Manual Handling	Infection Control
Apr				
May				
June				
July				
Aug				
Sept				
Oct				
Nov				
Dec				
Jan				
Feb				
March				

Orthotics	Induction	Fire	Manual Handling	Infection Control
Apr				
May				
June				
July				
Aug				
Sept				
Oct				
Nov				
Dec				
Jan				
Feb				
March				

Podiatry	Induction	Fire	Manual Handling	Infection Control
Apr				
May				
June				
July				
Aug				
Sept				
Oct				
Nov				
Dec				
Jan				
Feb				
March				

SLT	Induction	Fire	Manual Handling	Infection Control
Apr				
May				
June				
July				
Aug				
Sept				
Oct				
Nov				
Dec				
Jan				
Feb				
March				

Sickness Absence

Sickness Absence (%) Red > 5%, Amber 4% – 4.9%, Green < 4%, Target 4%

	Organisation	Directorate	Dietetics	O.T	Orthotics	Physio	Podiatry	SLT	Comments
Apr									
June									
July									
Aug									
Sept									
Oct									
Nov									
Dec									
Jan									
Feb									
Mar									

Sickness Absence (%)

Red > 5%, Amber 4% – 4.9%, Green < 4%, Target: Below 4%

	%	Directorate last 12 months	Organ. last 12 months	Directorate WTE days lost to stress/anxiety					

Staff Turnover (%)

Red >12%, Amber 10% -12%, Green <10%

Month	Budgeted WTE	Actual WTE (inc Overtime, bank, agency)	WTE Staff in Post	WTE Leavers	Directorate WTE Annual Turnover %	Organisation Annual Turnover %	Head Count in Post	Head Count Leavers	Space for Notes
Apr									
May									
June									
July									
Aug									
Sept									
Oct									
Nov									
Dec									
Jan									
Feb									
Mar									

Turnover Directorate Breakdown (%)

Red > 1% overspend, Amber < 1% overspend, Green 0% overspend, Target 0% or underspend

Budgeted WTE Month... Year...	Actual (worked inc bank/ agency) WTE Month... Year....	Variance (WTEs)	Cumulative pay budget (£000s)	Cumulative pay expend. (£000s)	Variance (£000s) Traffic Light	Monthly bankWTEs	Cumulative bank £s	Monthly agency WTEs	Cumulative agency £s	Cumulative overtime £s
Directorate										
Organisation										
WTEs										
Dietetics										
OT										
Orthotics										
Physio										
Podiatry										
SLT										
Total										

Template 17.3 Example AHP activity report

SERVICE ACTIVITY REPORT   DATE....................

MONTH	LAST FINANCIAL YEAR				THIS FINANCIAL YEAR				
	No. of Referrals	No. Face To Face Contacts	Below or Above Target for Month	Running Total for Year	No. of Referrals	% DNA	No. Face to Face Contacts	Below or Above Target for Month	Running Total for Year
APR									
MAY									
JUNE									
JULY									
AUG									
SEPT									
OCT									
NOV									
DEC									
JAN									
FEB									
MAR									
TOTALS									

Target for Year .... contacts.   Target for year ....referrals

First to Follow-up ratio for Year : ....

CHAPTER 18

Useful guidance

Robert Jones and Fiona Jenkins

USING TIME EFFECTIVELY

All managers and leaders occasionally waste time. However, the overall objective must be to eliminate non-value-added activities, thereby improving efficiency, effectiveness, and performance. In a recent survey undertaken by NHSI[1] significant areas of time wasing in management were identified.

- On average, leaders spend only 7.5% of time on planning, reflecting, and thinking.
- Of the average 54-hour week worked by an NHS manager, 38 hours were spent in meetings.
- Of the 26 meetings attended, only seven started on time.
- Only 36% of attendees actively participated in the meetings.

It may be worth considering other common time wasters we have listed here and how they might be minimised.

- Lack of written goals with deadlines.
- No plan with written checkpoints to assess progress.
- Inability to say 'no'.
- Deviating from the plan.
- Indecision—gathering information endlessly or gathering irrelevant information.
- Incomplete or poor information.
- Snap decisions based on insufficient evidence.
- Attempting too much at once.
- Resistance to making choices.
- Unwillingness or inability to delegate appropriately.
- Attempting too much by yourself—not accepting assistance or asking for help when legitimate and appropriate.

- Getting 'bogged down' with inappropriate details for the task.
- Failure to listen or take notes.
- Indifference or lack of motivation.
- Failure to break tasks into small, manageable parts.
- Lack of specific plans to meet goals selected.
- Lack daily priorities so that you don't know what to do first, second, and so on.
- Shifting priorities so you jump from one task to another.
- Crisis management arising from failure to plan for what could go wrong.
- Unrealistically low time estimates for the task.
- Interruptions; 'drop-in', unscheduled meetings.
- Personal disorganisation.
- Lack of self-discipline in staying with the project or piece of work until you get it done—not being a finisher.
- 'Red tape', paperwork, and bureaucracy.
- Writing papers that no one will read.
- Confused responsibility and authority.
- Not getting a clear rationale for what is required—managers/directors moving the goal posts.
- Inadequate equipment/facilities.
- Insufficient 'know-how' for particular tasks.
- Time spent looking for papers, poor filing system.
- Procrastination.

Box 18.1 Some tips for managing your time effectively

Consider the list above—do any of these apply to you?

Know your objectives and goals clearly—the ones you most need or want to reach.

Decide which activities are most important to achieving your objectives and goals.

Evaluate urgent-appearing work that comes your way; is it really urgent? Is it important? Can it wait until later? Does it require your attention or can you delegate it?

Handle the most valuable or important activities first. Let the quick, easy, less important things come later after you've achieved your main objectives for the day.

Make arrangements to avoid telephone interruptions when necessary.

Plan the diary to have 'drop-in' visitors.

Be sure of the remit with delegated tasks by manager/director.

Be sure to give clear remits for tasks you are giving to others.

Be sure information you are giving to others is correct.

Noise or visual distraction causes attention shift.

Take care planning meeting agendas so that agenda items have timings.

Restrict meetings to a set time span.

Start meetings on time.

Only have the relevant people to the business in hand.

Clarify responsibility, authority, and accountability.

Do not duplicate work or effort.

Do the task once only.

Ensure you have clear, relevant, timely, and accurate information.

Ensure appropriate training—time can be wasted because you do not 'know how'.

Ensure you have the necessary equipment or facilities.

Make sure your written work is accurate and do it only once.

Ensure you have some 'white space' in your diary; we all need time where the diary is 'clear'.

Keep your desk tidy—'untidy desk, untidy mind'!!

Work 'sensible' hours. Unreasonably long hours impact adversely on yourself, staff, and patients. Nobody is indispensible!

THE SEVEN PRINCIPLES OF PUBLIC LIFE

Box 18.2 The seven principles of public life

1 **Selflessness**. Holders of public office should take decisions solely in terms of the public interest. They should not do so in order to gain financial or other material benefits for themselves, their family, or their friends.

2 **Integrity.** Holders of public office should not place themselves under any financial or other obligation to outside individuals or organisations that might influence them in the performance of their official duties.

3 **Objectivity.** In carrying out public office, including making public appointments, awarding contracts, or recommending individuals for rewards and benefits, holders of public office should make choices on merit.

4 **Accountability.** Holders of public office are accountable for their decisions and actions to the public and must submit themselves to whatever scrutiny is appropriate to their office.

5 **Openness**. Holders of public office should be as open as possible about all the decisions and actions that they take. They should give reasons for their decisions and restrict information only when the wider public interest clearly demands.

6 **Honesty.** Holders of public office have a duty to declare any private inter-est relating to their public duties and to take steps to resolve any conflicts arising in any way that protects the public interest.

7 **Leadership.** Holders of public office should promote and support these principles by leadership and example.

'THE RULES THAT STIFLE CHANGE THAT <u>MUST</u> BE BROKEN'

1 Regard any new idea from below with suspicion.
2 Insist a hierarchy exists.
3 Criticise others' ideas.
4 Treat problems as a sign of failure.
5 Express criticisms; don't praise.
6 'Name and shame'.
7 Control everything.
8 Plan change in secret.
9 Delegate difficult decisions.
10 Count everything that moves ... frequently.

These are rules that definitely should be broken. From time to time, all of us will have been subjected to, or guilty of, one of these negative behaviours.

To be successful:

* make sure you are fit for purpose
* develop a vision
* value yourself
* ensure relevant roles for managers and leaders
* develop consultancy skills
* work together, respecting differences
* promote cross-boundary multidisciplinary and interdisciplinary working.

IS EVERYONE THE ARCHITECT OF THEIR OWN FUTURE?

AHP managers and leaders might consider their personal building blocks necessary for influencing future patterns of working. Perhaps the key aspirations listed in Box 18.3 are worthy of consideration.

Box 18.3 Key aspirations

1 Always ensure that patients are your top priority.
2 Hold onto the healthcare expertise and excellence you have striven for.
3 Be flexible, innovative, 'future proof', and be the solution not the problem.
4 Be business-minded, business-skilled, and business-'savvy', and aim to provide the service you would choose to use yourself.
5 Nurture, develop, and support your staff.
6 Keep costs under control; be responsible, but also entrepreneurial.
7 Look at your processes—can you do better?
8 Ensure AHPs work collaboratively; leave professional 'silos' behind.
9 Know and value yourself; hold onto your core values.
10 Demonstrate value for money, compete in the market place, and strive to be the best.

Index

Diagrams and drawings are given in italics

adult learning
  audit 117
  Brookfield's Principles of adult
    learning 112, 113
  complaints 116
  false stage 4 learners 111
  handovers 117
  importance of reflection 113–15, 118
  introduction 107–9
  models of reflection 114
  principles into practice 112–13
  resistant learners 111
  self-directed learners *115*
  significant event analyses/critical
    incident reporting 116–17
  SSDL model 111–12
  stages of development of *108–9*
  T1/S3-S4 mismatch 109–10
  T1/S4 mismatch 109
  T4/S1 mismatch 110–11
  work-based 113
algorithms 184, *185–6*
all-around flexible/adaptable teaching
  style 125
Allied Health Professions (AHP)
  management structures 2, 10, 31
  managers 2
'androgogy' 107
Anticipated Recovery Pathways (USA)
  174
assessment tool
  application 31–2

conclusions 33–4
example template *34–47*
introduction 31
scoring system 33
Audit Commission 176
audit research 75

Baker, A 133
balanced scorecards 7–8
BAPT *see* British Association for
  Psychological Type
Barsoux, J. 134
behavioural styles
  analysers 101–2, *103*
  category communication styles
    104–5, *104*
  directors 102, *103*, 105
  introduction 101
  relaters 102, *103*, 105
  socialisers 102, *103*, 105
  strengths and weaknesses 103
  teams 103–4
Belbin, R. Meredith 96
Belbin team role questionnaire 96–7,
  105
benchmarking tool
  briefing notes 50
  introduction 49–50
  section 1, general information 52
  section 2, professional group/
    staffing 52
  section 3, inpatient services 55

section 4, outpatient services 55, 57
section 5, community services 57, 59
spreadsheet 1 (organisation) *51*
spreadsheet 2 (professional group)
    53–4
spreadsheet 4 (outpatient services)
    56
spreadsheet 5 (community services)
    58
usage of 50
benefits realisation 6–7
Bennis, W. 134
big conference teaching style 125
BPM *see* business performance
    management
BPR *see* Business Process Re-engineering
Briggs, Katharine 78–9, 82
Bristow, J. 136
British Association for Psychological
    Type (BAPT) 87
Brookfield, S. D. 108
'bucket filling' (teaching) 126
Burgoyne, John 94
Burnes, Bernard 130, 132, 133
business performance management
    (BPM) 3
Business Process Re-engineering (BPR)
    133

Canadian Council on Health Services
    Accreditation 183
Carby, K. 136
care pathways
    aims of 176–8, *177*
    analysis 193
    benefits/barriers 194–5
    choosing a clinical area 178–9
    clinical governance 175–6
    collecting data 181–2
    conclusions 195–6
    contents 175
    description 172–4
    developing 174–5, 187–8, *188*
    documentation 191–2
    drafting 184–7, *187*
    evaluation 192, *193*
    introduction 171
    key indicators 183–4
    launching 188–91
    measurement 180–1
    reviewing current practice 182–3

reviewing the evidence 180
    ten phases 178
    use of 194
care planning 74
case study
    data/information 151–2
    evaluation 153–7
    introduction 150
    leadership skills 154
    learning points 157–8
    management skills 153–4
    managerial imperatives 151
    negotiation with stakeholders 152
    project groups 151
    setting direction 152
    shared vision 151
    specification phase 152
    staff participation 152
    triggers for change 150–1
change
    agent 138, *138*
    curve 138, *138*, 140
    eight-stage process of 138, *138*
    force field analysis 140, *140*
    iceberg process *139*, 140
    PDSA analysis 140–1, *141*
    PEST analysis *143*
    SWOT analysis 142, *142*
    time continuum *139*
change management
    case study *see* case study
    change 130–1
    communicating 143–4
    conclusions 158–60
    culture 133–4
    fatigue 144–5
    framework 148–9, *149–50*
    hierarchy of leadership 135
    introduction 129–30
    key behaviours 147–8
    key concepts 131–3
    key factors 146–7, *146–7*
    leadership 134–5, 144
    learning points 157–8
    models/techniques/approaches
        136–43, *137–8*
    overcoming change fatigue 144–5
    sigmoid curve 132, *132*
    teams 136
'Choice Appointments' 150, 153–5,
    158

clinical dashboard 7
computerised information systems
    data collection 71
    documentation 72
    hardware 70
    information use 70
    introduction 69
    reporting 71–2
    security 71
    service agreements 72
    software 70–1
    specific 70
    training 73

De Luc, K. 192
decision support 74
Deming, W. E. 5
dimensions
    E/I scale (energy) 80
    J/P scale (judging/perceiving) 82
    S/N scale (information) 81
    T/F scale (thinking/feeling) 81
DMAIC process 5
DNAs (did not attends) 150–1, 155–6, 155–7
document management 75
Domains 32–3

Eastbourne District General Hospital 150
European Pathway Association 173
Evidence-based medicine 173
extraverts 78, 80, 84–5

feeling 81–2, 85
'five whys' management technique 4
Freud, Sigmund 78

gastroenterology 50
general resource management 75
Gestalt-Field psychologists 132
Goleman, Daniel 135
Grow, G. 108, 110, 118, 125–6
guidance
    personal building blocks 228–9
    rules to be broken 228
    seven principles of public life 227–8
    time 225–7

handedness 79–80, 87
handwriting 79

Handy, Charles 132, 134
Health Professions Council 34
Hersey, Paul 108
Hirshhorn, L. 136
Hooper, A. 131–2, 135

Iles, V. 136
image management 75
information management
    functions for record systems 73–6
    introduction 73
Information Management and
    Technology (IM&T) 67, 69
INSEAD 1
Institute for Health Improvement
    European Forum (Prague) 158
Institute for Healthcare Improvement
    (USA) 182
Integrated Care Pathways (ICPs) 171-4,
    177–9, 183–4, 187–93, *188-9*, *193*,
    196-7, *see also* care pathways
International Web Portal 174
introverts 78, 80, 83–5
intuition 81, 85

Johnson, Samuel 130
Journal of Integrated Care 173
judging 82–3, 86
Jung, Carl 78–80, 81–2, 87

Kano Type 2 projects 158
Kaplan, Robert S. 8
Katzenbach J 136
key performance indicators (KPIs) 3
Knowles, M. S. 112
Kotter, J. 134
KPIs *see* key performance indicators

Langley, G. 182
Leadership Qualities Framework
    91, 94
lean thinking 3–4
Lewin, K. 133

McCalman, J. 146
McDonald, P. 197
McKee, L. 133
Management Quality Matrix (MQM)
    1–2, 8–10
Manager's Guide to Self-Development
    (Pedler/Burgoyne) 94

*Managing and Leading in the Allied
   Health Professions* (Eds-Jones/Jenkins)
   131
Map of Medicine 196
medicines management 75
metrics 2
Middleton, S. 193
Mintzberg, H. 135, 138, *138*
musculoskeletal problems 150
Myers, Isabel 78–9, 82
Myers-Briggs Type Indicator (MBTI)
      and 360° feedback 99
      background 78–9
      five scenarios 78
      four dimensions 80–7
      introduction 77
      taking forward 87
      type/preference 79–80

Nannus, B. 134
National Pathways Association (NPA)
   173
National Pathways User Group *see*
   National Pathway Association
NeLH pathways database 174
Next Stage Review 7
NHS Evidence 174, 179
NHSI Productive Series 4, 225
Nolan, K. 182
Nolan, T. 182
Norton, D. P. 8

Obholzer, A. 133
official curriculum teaching style 125
outcome indicators 183
outcome measurement
      community domiciliary 168–9
      inpatient services 167–8, *167–8*
      introduction 163–4
      outpatient services 164–7, *166–7*
Oxford Psychologists Press 87

PACS *see* picture archiving,
   communication system
patient contribution area 75
Patient Reported Outcome Measures
   (PROMS) 163
Patton, R. 146
PDSA cycles 182–3, *182*
Pedler, Mike 94
perceiving 82, 86

Perkins, D. 133
Pettigrew, F. 133
physiotherapy 50
picture archiving, communication
   system (PACS) 75
Pond, Christina 131
Potter, J. 131–2, 135
process indicators 183
professional groups 62
PROMS *see* Patient Reported Outcome
   Measures
Psychological Types (Jung) 78, 82

questionnaires 94, 105

receptive/non-receptive contexts for
   change 133
reports
      presentation 201–4
      writing 199–200
Roberts, A. 193
Roberts, V. 133
Rogers, Jenny 83
Roy, S. 171

Saunders, R. 143
Schein, E. 133–4
Schneider, S. 134
Schon, D. 133
schools of thought
      group dynamic 132
      individual perspective 132
      open systems 132
screening 74
Self-Directed Learning model (SSDL)
   108, 111–12, *112*, 125–8
sensing 81, 83, 85
sensitive, student centred teaching style
   125
SETS *see* Staffordshire Evaluation of
   Teaching Styles (SETS)
Shaper role 97
Six Sigma 4–5
SMART 181
Smith, D. 136
SNOMED *see* Systematised
   Nomenclature of Medicine
SSDL *see* Self-Directed Learning model
staff activity
      implementation 62
      introduction 61–2

part 1, general information 62–3
part 2, patient-related activity 63
part 3, non patient-related activity 63–4
part 4, contracted hours/caseload 64
reports from activity sample 65, 66–7
summary 67
therapy services activity sample *pro forma* 64–5
Staffordshire Evaluation of Teaching Styles (SETS) 120, 126
stages of learning
   1 108–11, 127–8
   2 108, 127–8
   3 108, 127–8
   4 108, 111, 127–8
Standards
   1 strategy 10, *10–11*
   2 patient and service user experience *11–12*
   3 clinical excellence *13–14*
   4 finance *14–16*
   5 information and metrics *16–17*
   6 activity *17–18*
   7 staff resources *19–20*
   8 staff management, education, development *20–1*
   9 service improvement and redesign *21–3*
   10 leadership and management development *23–4*
   11 risk management *24–5*
   12 corporate governance *25–6*
   13 communication and marketing *26–7*
   14 top five key performance indicators *28*
   Management Quality overall action plan *28*
   record of Standard completion/ review dates *29*
straight facts, no-nonsense teaching style 125
stress 86–7
strokes *188–9*
structure indicators 183
Sutherland, K. 136
Systematised Nomenclature of Medicine (SNOMED) 75

teaching styles
   awareness 119
   choice 124
   delivery/various styles *125*
   introduction 119–20
   investigating 120–1, *121–4*
   matching 124–6
   providing methods of learning 125
   recursive 127–8
   and stages of learning 126
teamwork 86
templates
   activity report *224*
   clinical governance *206–14*
   human resources performance report *215–23*
terminology 75
Thakur, M. 136
thinking 81, 82, 85
360° feedback
   briefing respondents 95–6
   description 89–90
   feedback grid *98*
   follow up 99
   gathering 92–3
   in practice 91–2
   questions 93–5
   receiving 97–9
   use of 90–1
   using other instruments 96–7
   who to ask 95
Total Quality Management (TQM) 5–6, 133
Toyota 3
TQM *see* Total Quality Management
tracking 74
traffic light scoring mechanism 32–3, *32*
traits 79
types
   ENFP 83–4
   ISTJ 83–4

value difference 79

Wesley F. 135, 138, *138*
Wilson, J. 173
workflow management 74
WTE
   non-registered staff 59
   registered staff 59
'WYSIWYG' personality 80